ISBN: 978-0-993470011

First published in the UK in 2015
Second edition published in the UK in 2019
by:
Seeking Sense and Science Ltd.
Bluebell Cottage, High Street, Stroud, GL6 8DR

    https:www.facebook.com/marinayoung.aquestforwellbeing/
Email address: seekingsenseandscience@gmail.com

To my parents:
For their patience and enthusiasm. For listening to me for hours as I verbalised and consolidated all I was reading and discovering, and for their robust questioning.

To my husband:
For his patience and for helping me to have the time to embark on my journey of discovery.

To my daughter:
For being careful not to eat too much sugar.
I hope this book will give her a head start for an energetic, healthy and happy life.

Page

FOREWORD

I Want To Break With Tradition ……

I would like to start with presenting some of the golden nuggets of this book as early on as possible because, there is a danger, today, that we are drowning in the written and spoken word. So many books and blogs, so much chatter on tv and the internet. With all the misinformation and poor science mixed in, arriving at any useful conclusion is becoming increasingly hard.

My Journey In And Out Of Rheumatoid Arthritis

This book covers many topics but I am particularly excited by some of the information I have found because I see that it is greatly responsible for providing very positive results for many people, including my own journey in and out of Rheumatoid Arthritis. The regained health, mental clarity, weight loss, reduction in pain and suffering that is taking place, in some quarters, across the world compels me to ensure an important message is not being lost in all the conflicting noise.

I Want The Prospect Of A Good Old Age

We are living longer, but with what prospects? Can we not have a higher expectation of mental and physical agility into old age? The message is 'yes we can'. More than three quarters of our western woes, including heart disease, strokes, chronic diseases, cancers and weight issues, can be significantly avoided through a better understanding of our master hormone, insulin. A central player, that has been, almost entirely, ignored and misunderstood.

The Secret To Becoming And Staying Slim

Weight loss is slow, difficult and often unsuccessful without basic knowledge of insulin, a master switch to energy, fat storage and our hunger and satiety hormones. Failure to lose weight and gain health has very little to do with calories but everything to do with being fed a lot of misinformation.

*Be 'insulin savvy' and you can take command of your health and your weight …
and slow down the speed at which you age.*[1]

Why We Should See Ourselves Like Hybrid Cars

We should be equally excited about the science that is showing us that we will do well if we run our bodies like hybrid cars, as we were designed to.

A Fuel For Enhanced Performance

In this book I explore the fact that we evolved to run on two fuels but many in the west are running, predominantly, on one. We should be in a state of burning fat for fuel far, far more often than we are. The benefit, when we do is not to be underestimated, for fat is a 'clean' fuel that produces ketones in our body, enhancing our physical and mental performance. When we burn body fat we also help regenerate and repair our body as well.

A Fuel That Makes Us Age Faster

Alarmingly, however, we chose to fill our tanks with a fuel that impairs our performance, producing a lot of unwanted 'smoke' in the form of free radicals and oxidative stress, speeding up our ageing process and making us ill. The fuel that we burn most of the time is sugar, in the form of simple sugars and low fibre, grain based foods.

Paying Attention to Positive Patient Outcomes

A growing section of the scientific, medical and nutritional world is proposing a major reversal of long existing advice on food. This is resulting in exciting levels of positive patient outcomes (including the reversal of my own illness) and increased mental and physical agility at all ages. It is this positive patient outcome and improvement of the overall health of the people who have adopted the new nutritional approaches that compels me to write about it, with a desire to replace confusion with a fresh sense of hope and purpose.

My Story – Briefly

In 2009 I was diagnosed with Rheumatoid Arthritis. For 3 years I was prescribed steroids and told to stay on immuno-suppressants for life. Not happy to live in this potential "bio-chemical chaos" that led onto anti-depressants, I wanted to learn why I had RA. Could finding the cause eliminate the need for medication?

Why Should You Read What I Have To Say?

I have spent 10 years researching. Reading countless books and scientific papers courtesy of Google Scholar. Through the magic of the internet, I have been privileged enough to "attend" thousands of hours of scientific and medical lectures, conferences and interviews, all over the world.

My quest for knowledge has been obsessive and has coincided with extremely exciting times in this area of evolving science. This has, undoubtedly, been driven by the advent of the internet and the incredible volume of exchange of information. The on-line world has enabled alternative thinkers to meet outside of the 'scientific establishment' who traditionally maintain a tight grip on change and new thinking.

Planning World Take-Over At 92

Growing up, I was strongly influenced by my father. He worked from home and innovated and developed technology in a number of different industries. With a degree in chemical engineering from Imperial College, London, he is an avid reader and researcher. Annoyingly, when I was growing up, he was very partial to extensive monologues (that hasn't changed)! At 92, he is following my approach towards nutrition and busy planning world domination with all his various projects!

A Critical Attitude Towards All Information

Without realising it, listening to him all those years, I was taking in information on many topics but more importantly I was absorbing an attitude towards information. Questioning and scientific reasoning were relentlessly drummed into me.

I have noticed that the more scientifically trained an individual is, the less they are likely to talk in absolute terms. As soon as you think you have the answer, you have to keep questioning. Beware of emphatic phrases! Though I am sure I am guilty of them myself ....

So much of what I have read has been buried in books and long articles that most may not have the time or inclination to navigate, not to mention the thousands of hours of lectures that I have listened to. I hope, therefore, that more people may also have the chance to share my interesting journey by reading this book.

Finally Free of Medication
I have been medication-free since 2013, I don't even take paracetamol. I feel healthier than I have felt in years.

Advice that Leads to Much Suffering
Since the era of food guidelines, a medicating approach to illness and an institutional, rigid, consensus on medical advice, we have experienced an ever-worsening level of chronic disease in the West. Although we are living longer we are seeing increased levels of suffering in old age, especially with dementia and late stage gut dysfunction and cancers.

A Launch Pad to a Lifetime of Good Questions
Whether it be the conflict of information over heart health, how truly toxic sugar is, how confused we have become about dietary fat or discovering that the topic of gut bacteria is as complex as the study of the Universe, I hope you will view each topic as a launch pad for you to pursue and question. When seeking new individuals or sources, make sure, as much as possible, that their observations are unhindered by the prospect of profit or promotion.

All facets of health and nutrition are evolving, interconnected stories with no definitive ending (certainly not in our lifetime). As science discovers answers it immediately throws up more questions.

A Who's Who Of New Thinkers
The "Further Recommended Reading" at the end of this book is a Who's Who of some brilliant minds, across the world, all in communication with each other and pushing ahead, finding real solutions for many. Through their new understanding of nutrition and how our body responds to good and bad foods they are enabling more and more positive patient outcomes.

So Keep An Open Mind, Even on the Things You Believe to be Right
The more knowledge is gained the more amazing we find the relationship between nutrition and our body and the more we have to acknowledge how little we know. We must always keep questioning, even the things that seem right to us now.
We are all students forever …..

THE NUGGETS THAT SHOULDN'T BE BURIED

Nugget Number 1

We evolved to run on two fuels but too many run on only one

This fact:
- **Is at the root of our suffering**
- **Speeds up our ageing and**
- **Leaves us with poor prospects of a good old age**

Fat or thin many of us in the west are in trouble. Our prospects for a physically and mentally agile old age are not good. We evolved to regularly burn fat to fuel our bodies. (1) Yet today in the West we mostly burn sugar for fuel.

Weight gain, inflammatory disease including heart disease and rapid ageing are driven by too much carbohydrate (not just sugar). Healthy fats are not to blame.

Nugget Number 2

Sugar is a "dirty" fuel that creates oxidation
Burning sugar for fuel too frequently reduces mental performance and
Leads to a faster mental and physical decline

Even if we have successfully cut sugar from our diet, we are eating too frequently and too many grain based foods. The negative consequences of this are being dramatically overlooked but equally dramatically felt.

Nugget Number 3

Fat is a "clean" fuel
When we burn fat we produce ketones

When glucose from carbohydrates is in short supply, the body will burn fat and produce ketones. The brain cannot burn fat so the body converts the fat to ketones that are then used as fuel by the brain. As the body can only store carbohydrate for one or two days, the brain would shut down if it were not for ketones. If ketones are present, the brain will spare the glucose and take up the ketones as the preferred fuel for the brain (1a).

Nugget Number 4

When the body produces ketones it is in a state of ketosis
There are many benefits to ketosis

To be in ketosis significantly fewer low fibre carbohydrates can be consumed such as bread, pasta and rice. Plenty of high fibre carbohydrates such as vegetables can still be consumed. Ketones are produced from either burning body fat (if weight loss is desired) or otherwise healthy dietary fat. An increase of healthy fats in the diet is beneficial as this enables the body to be in ketosis leading to significantly higher mental and physical endurance.[1b]

Benefits of Ketosis:
- It can improve overall health
- Hunger is reduced
- Weight loss is easy
- Reduction in inflammation, prevention and reversal of inflammatory diseases
- Type 2 diabetes can be reversed
- A powerful tool in preventing and fighting cancer
- Helps reduce anxiety and depression[2]
- Studies are showing that it may help to resolve migraine
- Epilepsy has been controlled by ketosis for many years, even without drugs
- Helps improve acne
- It can help improve menstrual problems
- It can help combat infertility

Nugget Number 5

The body can not burn fat until sugar, stored in the liver, is depleted (around 8-12 hours supply)

Our western diet, full of sugar and low fibre, grain-based foods, combined with eating too frequently is preventing us from burning fat for fuel for much of the time. Yet when we burn fat for fuel we are better set to benefit from:
- More energy
- Better mental clarity[2a]
- A slowing down of the ageing process and an
- Immune system and inflammatory response that remains IN CONTROL.

10

Nugget Number 6
The new buzz word is "inflammageing"
Sugar burners lose control of their inflammation "off switch" *(3)*
Our immune system acts like the welcoming committee from hell (to borrow a rather graphic phrase from Cancer Research UK). Working to protect us from foreign invaders, be they toxins, viruses, bacteria, or the ravages of an unhealthy lifestyle. It sends white blood cells to attack invaders with brutal force. This powerful attack is known as an *inflammatory response* but needs to be over quickly in order to minimise damage to healthy tissue. The need to speedily shut down this process should not be underestimated.

Nugget Number 7

Inflammation is dragging many towards disease
The inability to switch off the inflammatory response is slowly dragging many, in varying degrees, in western society, towards disease, pain and mental decline. It is at the core of most of our western illnesses, including type 2 diabetes, heart disease, the different forms of arthritis, many allergies, asthma and cancer.

Regular sugar burners will also suffer:
- Brain fog
- Lethargy
- Weight issues
- Hormonal imbalances

Nugget Number 8
There are two ways of burning fat
Either through fasting or from consuming a higher fat, low carbohydrate diet

Burning Body Fat
Burning off stored sugar (glycogen) in the liver during fasting will enable you to tap into your stored body fat to produce ketones. This will enable successful weight loss.

Burning Dietary Fat
Increasing dietary fat and keeping carbohydrate consumption low (plenty of vegetables can still be consumed) will allow the body to burn fat consumed in the diet enabling the body to produce ketones.

Nugget Number 9

The understanding of cholesterol is being turned on its head.
A good cholesterol ratio can be achieved by increasing intake of saturated
fat and reducing intake of low carbohydrates, especially sugar and grains.

Consumption of healthy fats, including saturated fats allows for a more efficient flow of food energy. Low fibre carbohydrates, even in small, frequent quantities disrupt our hunger and fat storage hormones in a way that hinders the efficient flow of energy through our body. This can eventually lead to higher triglycerides (fat) in the blood. See Chapter 9

Nugget Number 10

Our bodies should be metabolically flexible or 'fat adapted'
So that we can easily switch between
Burning fat and burning glucose (sugar) for fuel

Are You 'Fat Adapted?'

Many people are permanent sugar burners for whom running out of sugar fuel is too uncomfortable to ignore; compelling them to consume more sugar or carbohydrates. A little knowledge of our master hormone insulin enables a clearer understanding of what we must do to regain or maintain health.

Nugget Number 11

Better understanding and education can
Prevent and reverse so much suffering

The prospect of eventual weight gain in youth and dementia, inflammatory pain and disease in old age can be substantially prevented by understanding how to adapt to burning fat more frequently than most of us do today. This includes the ability to achieve and maintain weight loss.

Nugget Number 12

Insulin - mastering our master hormone
Knowing how to control insulin is the biggest step we can take to
Mastering our weight, health and good prospects into old age[5]
The length of our life is regulated by insulin.

Nugget Number 13

Insulin's nickname is 'the fat storage hormone'. Constantly triggering insulin and not allowing it to subside never allows fat burning

Sugar and low fibre carbs significantly trigger the release of insulin in the blood. Insulin is critical to many vital mechanisms including stable blood sugars. Yet insulin is responsible for storing fat. The more sugars and grain based foods we eat, the more we trigger insulin and the more fat we will store. For, in nature, insulin is vital for storing nutrients in times of plenty so that nutrients are available when times are hard. For us, today, the supply of food is unlimited and continuous.

Nugget Number 14

Stored fat can be visible fat or invisible
In some thin people, fat can be stored, dangerously,
Around the major organs

Fat cells differ considerably from person to person depending on their genes. This is why a very small percentage of the clinically obese remain healthy whilst many outwardly thin people become ill with obesity related conditions. (4)

Nugget Number 15

Fat cells do not sit idle
They are busy signalling, or, more importantly
Can disrupt signalling with the rest of the body

Fat or thin, the more insulin we stimulate, the more fat we store and the more we over-produce pro-inflammatory signals. It is this simple fact that, over time, leads to many of our illnesses, including heart disease and strokes.

Nugget Number 16

Chronic (non-stop), silent inflammation can go largely undetected for years.
It is at the core of our failing health and weight gain

Inflammation is at the root of most of our issues in the gut, in the joints, in the arteries and many other of our countless chronic diseases that we suffer from in the west. Cancer, too, can be factored into this disruptive process.

Nugget Number 17

Hyperinsulinemia (stimulating too much insulin)
Leads to inflammation

Nugget Number 18

Too much insulin leads us to become less sensitive to insulin
That unfortunately leads our body to pump out even more insulin
Creating a vicious cycle

The more insulin we trigger through frequently eating the wrong foods, the less efficient insulin becomes in doing its job - But insulin MUST get sugar into our cells and out of the blood. So the pancreas responds by making even more insulin. Yes, it gets the job done and sugar is moved to the cells but it further increases insulin's inefficiency. This inefficiency is known as *insulin resistance.*

Nugget Number 19

Today insulin resistance is starting in childhood;
Its adverse effects, normally associated with the elderly,
Are being seen in ever-younger people
Yet insulin resistance is not even on our radar?

Unfortunately insulin and inflammation have been like a horse and cart(5a) but with little clarity as to "who was driving whom" and things were not helped by a bit of bad timing in science....

Nugget Number 20

The timing of science led type 2 diabetes to be viewed as a disease of blood sugar instead of a disease of blood insulin

Unluckily the ability to measure blood sugar levels and cholesterol were discovered before the technique to measure insulin resistance. If these discoveries had been in reverse order, we may have viewed *hyperinsulinemia* (too much insulin) and insulin resistance as the major contributors to heart disease, not cholesterol. (5b)

14

Unstoppable Momentum
Unfortunately the massive juggernaut of health care and vested interest created to deal with conditions such as heart disease and stroke, amongst others, had built up too much momentum to stop and turn back to revise our approach to heart disease and type 2 diabetes.

Type 2 Diabetes Starts Out as a Disease of Too Much Insulin
Even type 2 diabetes would have been treated differently and could have been caught years earlier.(5) For type 2 diabetes is a disease of too much insulin from too much insulin-stimulating foods.(6) High blood sugar is a "late stage symptom" as the over-production of insulin can continue to disguise the disease for years by forcing glucose into the cells thus maintaining stable blood sugars. All the while, it is insulin itself that leads the way to the slow build up of arterial and tissue damage that causes heart disease and stroke.(7) Yet it is not being monitored because no one is looking for hyperinsulinemia.

The Tragically Ignored Majority Player
Hyperinsulinemia (caused by eating too many foods that trigger too much insulin) is obviously not at the root of *all* disease but it is a majority player in much of our western woes. So much so that we would surely make a significant impact on the level of disease and suffering if we were to address it properly, both medically (through diet, actually) and through education. Some scientists go as far as saying that hyperinsulinemia and the weight problems it can cause leading to chronic inflammation could account for 80% of our health issues!

The age-old practice of fasting and better understanding of food groups
can prevent and reverse insulin resistance
where simple caloric restriction has failed
It is not just about calories in, calories out. It is about hormones, it is about insulin.

If You Think About It … What Do We Feed Babies to Put Weight On Fast?
The answer is of course, milk. A mother's milk is the only source in nature where high levels of fat are found in combination with high sugar (lactose). A baby needs to gain weight fast. The lactose (carbohydrate) in milk stimulates production of insulin (fat storage hormone) and in its presence enables the high level of fat in the milk to be quickly pushed to fat deposits in the baby's body. In addition a mother's milk contains ketones allowing the rapid development of the baby's brain. (8)

How This Affects Us
For us, fats and sugars (carbohydrates) are the worst combination of foods to eat with regards to fat accumulation for exactly this reason. Sugar triggers the fat storage hormone (insulin) so the fat and excess sugar energy we eat goes straight to our fat cells to be stored. … Those lovely, frothy cappuccinos are not a good start to the day.

The Power of Reversing Illness Through Fasting and Good Fats
The rediscovered art of intermittent fasting and understanding of the benefits of a higher amount of quality fat in the diet, coinciding with a meaningful reduction in low fibre carbohydrates has been part and parcel of many people's success in reacquiring insulin sensitivity leading to less insulin circulating in the blood. Those who have pursued this strategy have achieved good health and enhanced physical and mental performance. It has taken courage in these individuals to go against the high carb, low fat mantra that has been official advice since the 1970s.
Understanding insulin reveals much more starkly a major enemy….

A Nemesis that Takes Us Captive and Kills Us Slowly
Though glucose in sugar and carbohydrates, as well as stress and poor sleep have affected our health throughout the ages, due also to their effect on insulin; today we have another nemesis that has speeded up our insulin dysfunction, and therefore, our ageing process. It has reduced our quality of life and caused much suffering and premature death. It is not a new enemy but its army has expanded beyond comprehension and it is everywhere, like at no other time in the age of man. It takes us captive and kills us slowly …..
Who is This Enemy?
                    Its name is FRUCTOSE

16

We have severely underestimated how toxic sugar is
In the quantities we have consumed it in and
In particular how much more dangerous fructose is compared to glucose

Do Not Be Fooled By Its Disguise

We associate fructose as a natural, healthy sugar but only in moderate and infrequent amounts, consumed in whole fruits with fibre. We cannot say that just because something is "natural", it is healthy. There are many toxins in nature.

Table Sugar: Sucrose Is Made Up Of: 50% Fructose + 50% Glucose

Fructose is much sweeter than glucose and for many years has been used in concentrated amounts in processed foods, both sweet and savoury.

Fructose Speeds Up the Ageing Process (9)

The impact of fructose's burden on the liver should not be underestimated. Fructose can only be metabolised in 1.5kg of liver tissue whereas glucose is metabolised in the whole body (about 70kgs worth of body tissue in an average person). Yet fructose accounts for 50% of sugar's load. Insulin behaves differently in different organs and, in the liver, insulin resistance develops at an alarming rate. It is insulin dysfunction that ultimately leads to the blood sugar issues in type 2 diabetes. It drives cancer and it is the road to heart disease and strokes. The amount of sugar, and therefore fructose, that our children have access to today is why we are seeing younger people falling victim to these illnesses.

"Don't Eat Between Meals" …. Remember That Concept?

In the past, the **much smaller quantities** of sugar (thus fructose) consumed and little to no snacking meant that type 2 diabetes was less common and would occur at a much later age and so was referred to as "age on-set diabetes".

Fructose Goes By Many Names

Fructose may be labelled: natural corn syrup, isolated fructose, maize syrup, glucose/fructose syrup, tapioca syrup and more. Whatever its form, even in ordinary table sugar or in frequent, daily consumption of fruit, fructose works in a unique way in our body that can lead us to serious problems … and it does.

Fructose is Addictive, Disruptive and Everywhere (10)

Know our enemy and we stand a chance. If you don't think you consume much of it, think again. Fructose in fruit is obtainable all year round and is viewed as a "healthy snack" between meals. Fructose is put in everything from canned drinks, sports drinks, fruit juice, sweet food, savoury food, sweet sauces and savoury sauces but, unlike glucose, it also disrupts our hormones extremely quickly. We do not need much on a regular basis, year round, for it to set in motion the process of insulin resistance. A process that continues to be fuelled, and made worse, by glucose in the carbohydrates we eat, and in the frequency we consume them.

Fructose is a Life Saver in the Animal Kingdom

Fructose is truly toxic in the amount we eat and it is addictive. It leads us to feel hungry all the time, never allows a feeling of fullness and disrupts signals to our brain that tell us we have plenty of fat stored. This lack of signal leads our brain to think that we are starving, inclining us to slow down and conserve our energy. In other words, it leads to the lethargy and tiredness that so many sugar addicts experience. In Chapter 10, 'Sugar Unwrapped', we will discover why these seemingly toxic characteristics are a lifesaver in the Animal Kingdom.

The Ingredient At The Core Of Our Suffering ….

Understanding the destructive power of fructose, the extent of its presence in our lives, and how quickly it can set in motion problems, will substantially reduce our likelihood of obesity, chronic disease, heart disease, cancer and dementia.

… And At the Core of Our Ageing

The more sugars we have circulating around our body over our lifetime, the faster we will age. (11) Through a process called *glycation,* we essentially, slowly, caramelise over time! You cannot stop it but you can slow it down. Through glycation, sugar and protein molecules merge to form tough and inflexible tissue, leading to, not only, wrinkled skin but "wrinkled" internal organs as well, creating a lack of flexibility and functionality in the internal workings of the body. This unpleasant process needs to be significantly reduced if we wish to age well. In today's society, the good news is – we have *a lot of room for improvement!*

WHY WEIGHT LOSS HAS BEEN SO HARD FOR SO MANY PEOPLE?

The Problem
Established theory has said that: **Excess Weight Leads To Insulin Resistance**. So to lose weight we do NOT focus on insulin because it is seen as a result of weight gain, not a cause. This leads us to need to find another reason for weight gain. The conclusion promoted heavily over the last century has been that weight gain is caused by excess calories and not enough exercise. Not surprisingly the solutions have lead to repeated failure for many, as they pounded the treadmills at the gym, making themselves hungry whilst simultaneously eating small amounts of carbohydrates, leading to a permanent state of hunger.

Success with a New Approach
Success for many has been achieved by pursuing, almost, the exact opposite to the theory above and that is: **Too Much Insulin Leads to Excess Weight.** (12.) Unlike the first theory, if too much insulin causes weight gain then we need to examine what causes too much insulin – we cannot just ignore it. Yet it has been ignored, even in general practice, unless a person has been diagnosed as diabetic.
We will examine further on in the book how improving our sensitivity to insulin can easily achieve and maintain weight loss.

A Heavy and Mysterious Curtain
It would appear that so much of the suffering that is being experienced is unnecessary and can be reversed with a little bit more understanding. The medical community has mystified medicine, giving ailments unfathomable latin labels, telling us to listen to the doctors without question, and putting the beauty and elegance of how our body works behind a dark, heavy and mysterious curtain. Yet, we can all have a fundamental understanding of how our bodies work. We must understand because, when we do, we are far more likely to do the right thing and become healthier and slimmer.

So these are not just words …. This is what is happening
To our loved ones, to our children, to us
The positive side is that in so many cases,
We can do so much more for ourselves, than our doctors can do for us ….
If we take responsibility.

CHAPTER **1** :   WHERE WE ARE TODAY

Where We Are Today

- Overfed and undernourished
- Confused and misinformed
- Over medicated and overweight
- Intoxicated
- Suffering chronic body inflammation
- Suffering weakened immunity
- Disconnected from our bodies
- Forgotten basic knowledge for better nutrition and health
- Facing chronic disease
- Illness and
- Mental decline

Where We Could Be

- Lean and toned
- Energetic and focused
- Happy and calm
- Healthy
- Mentally agile
- Less fretful of disease
- Higher expectations of well-being into old age
- Better informed
- We could be thriving instead of just surviving

*There are two common characteristics found
in people who live over 100 years of age.
One is high cholesterol(2) and second is a low insulin status.(3)*

Distracted by Cholesterol
It would appear that longevity, on-going health, weight issues and long-term mental performance can be measured in a blood test … yet most have never had this marker checked.(3) Whilst we have been focused for so many decades on cholesterol, have we missed the true culprit, insulin?

Understanding how to regulate insulin is so important and easy. Yet knowledge has been ignored and a vital message continues to be lost to many.

Can We Become Less Fretful Of Disease And Mental Decline?
Yes, we can but, unfortunately all the conflicting noise and vested interest has led, up until now, it would seem, to unnecessary suffering.

How Are We Suddenly Curing The Incurable?
How is it that "incurable" type 2 diabetics are suddenly being cured and people who have fought for decades with weight issues are suddenly experiencing fast and permanent weight loss? Yet at the same time, obesity, diabetes and chronic diseases are on the rise and we still have stubbornly poor prospects for cancer and heart disease.

Why? What's going on? I hope to be able to cut through some of this confusion and give a revealing overview of the complete u-turn being made by more and more people in the world of health and nutritional science.

Who is right? Who is wrong?
Vegan. Vegetarian. Paleo. Ketogenic. Carnivore. Calorie restriction. Intermittent fasting. These are significantly different ways of fuelling our bodies. Which should we follow … if any, and why?

Why Should Governments Advise Us on Diet?

The very concept of government issuing a food guideline in the first place is questionable. Governments generally do not have good track records at getting things right! So why should we ever have trusted them to have the final say on diet? Who is advising them what to say? How much does lobbying and money affect governments' conclusions? Change in policies are slow and our health can not afford to wait.

Time to Offer Hope

There are people from all the disciplines of the scientific community coming together to bring a more rigorous scientific approach to the topic of health. There are also many doctors firmly devoted to this revolution for they are on the frontline of ill health. They are fed up with promoting and advising treatments that have done little more than patch the symptoms of illness, offering little hope of cure and well-being.

We Must Not Let Good Science Be Obscured by Dogma

The way so called "scientific" research is organised and funded today in established circles needs to be severely criticised and reformed. Vested interest is too corrupting to allow good science to surface, so good science is often obscured or dropped. Additionally, peer review of scientific papers leads to pressure to toe the line on existing dogma. New thinking that undermines old thinking may not result in good promotion prospects!

Speaking Out

In January 2009, Dr Marcia Angell, a former Editor-in-Chief of The New England Journal of Medicine, arguably the most important medical journal in the world, was quoted in The New York Review of Books:

"It is no longer possible to trust much of the clinical research that is published or to rely on the judgement of trusted physicians or authoritative medical guidelines. I take no pleasure in this conclusion which I reached slowly and reluctantly over my two decades as an Editor of The New England Journal of Medicine."

Has a Spell Been Broken?

As for the rest of us – has a spell been broken? We were once all much greater believers in the power of the magic bullet created in pharmaceutical laboratories – tablets and pills to fix everything. But at what price? Yes, we are living longer, but in what shape and with what prospects? Common sense may be prevailing over the reliance on false promises.

Decades of Slumber

The discussion of what has happened to food is becoming more sophisticated and more interesting than it has ever been. People are waking up from a slumber that has lasted several decades, during which time we have lost control of our food and relied too heavily on more and more pills. Those that have fully awoken now understand how truly toxic sugar is and how it, together with too many carbohydrates, are driving cancer.

Taking Responsibility for Ourselves

This book is about taking our health into our own hands and embarking on fact-finding missions to decide for ourselves what is right and what is wrong, for we may well be following the wrong advice.

Epigenetics

Until recently we were led to believe that the DNA we are born with predetermined our health and illnesses; that having certain genes would make it inevitable that, sooner or later, they would kick in and we would become ill.

Today we have cause to feel far more empowered and in control of our health. We are discovering, through a science known as "Epigenetics" [1], that the food we eat and the lifestyles we choose to lead have a direct effect on how the vast majority of our genes behave. By controlling our metabolism (the amount, type and frequency of energy taken in through food), we can maintain healthier cells and rid ourselves of cells containing broken and faulty genes.

Within A Whisper Of Triggering Illness

The power we have over our health through what we put in our mouths should not be underestimated – the good choices and the bad ones.

We overdo it, don't get enough sleep, eat badly and are within a whisper of triggering illness … but re-establishing a healthy routine with an eye on food, sleep, exercise and stress can not only keep us on the path of good health but restore health as well.

Answers With Added Value
If my experience is anything to go by, in the end I did find answers to my illness and along the way I found improvement and solutions to many other aspects of my poor health, including:
More energy
No more mood swings
No more anxiety
Better concentration
Better skin
Weight-loss
Better sleep and waking up refreshed

I rediscovered a sense of calm, energy and achievement. For it would seem that when you heal, you heal your whole body …. it is not a selective process.

Black Holes And Flat Earthers
Taking responsibility for ourselves means self-education; a privilege more available to us today through the internet. However the internet is a mix of incredible access to knowledge but potentially a black hole to information as there is so much of it and often very conflicting.

So we need to be wary of 'facts'. We have been dished up so many over the years that then go on to be overturned.

We need to question everything and be mindful when finding the same fact repeated endlessly; it does not make it necessarily true. It is essential to go back to basics.

As self-educators the trick, often, is finding the right questions to ask and being mindful of how the questions are posed. For example: Why are potatoes good for us? Or why are potatoes bad for us? Can lead you down two very different routes.

The whole subject of health is in such a state of flux, disagreement and confusion. In fact, it shows us that it is still possible for scientific opinion to be as divided and dogmatic as it was at the time when some believed the world to be flat and others round. Fat, protein, carbohydrates and opinions on whole grains are examples of where fervent, 'religious' division can lie.   Everything is being questioned.

Great Expectations
I suppose we would start with trying to eat our "five a day" but we have deviated so far down a road of poor and harmful eating habits that we are expecting those well travelled five little fruits and veg to accomplish rather a lot!

Opening Our Minds To A Bigger Picture
We need to stand back and look at a much bigger picture to understand what is impacting on our well-being and even our weight. We need to pay attention to the effects of medication, environmental toxins, stress, sleep and eating habits because they are having far more significant consequences on our bodies than we may have realised.

Our Daily Chemical Exposure
For example how many 'bottles' of products do you have in your house? In your kitchen? It seems you need at least five different products just for your dishwasher! In your bathroom? Cleaning, washing, cosmetics, grooming … we are sold substance after substance by the marketing men. Our bodies are dealing with more chemicals than ever before.

Remember, whatever we put on our skin goes straight into our bloodstream, let's try to keep that in mind! How long has that moisturizer been sitting on the shelf … indeed, what are those preservatives doing in your blood stream! What other chemicals are we subjected to in our home and work environments; in our cars and in all the goods that we purchase? Even the till receipts turn out to be cancerous! … And we top it all with mountains of medication.

I'm No Earth Mother But …

I don't think anyone I know would describe me as an "Earth mother". Yet my journey of discovery has led me to realise that we need to claw back a closeness to nature in every way we can, in a world that is moving in the opposite direction. We did not evolve to exist in the chemical, plastic, antiseptic, sprayed environment we live in today, removed from nature, fresh, fresh food and limited exposure to sunlight and soil.

Reconnecting with the Bacterial World

There is a balance that we have lost between protecting ourselves from, and interacting with, the bacterial world around us.

When we are exposed to bacteria we pick up the good and the bad. If we feed ourselves correctly, we feed the good bacteria what it needs. This will enhance our immunity and protect us from the bad bacteria that we are inevitably exposed to as well. So through exposure and good eating habits, we can build up our immune systems and be strong. Instead we have sterilised our immediate environments, sealed the windows, chosen to consume poor food and become weak.

Our bodies work flat out to metabolise and 'deal' with the chemicals that we let in, through medication, cosmetics, junk food, pollution, plastics, chemicals and the electro-magnetic frequencies emanating from our phones. The ammunition that our bodies need to counteract this assault takes the form of minerals, vitamins and polyphenol phytonutrients and fibre available from wholefoods, fresh vegetables, good quality protein and healthy fats.

So we must eat well not only to have the nutrients we need to enhance our bacterial immunity but also to protect us from the external assault of chemicals and toxins and finally with what goodness is left over to enable our bodies to function well so that we, in turn, can feel well, energetic and happy.

Can We Not Adapt More Intelligently to the World Around Us?

Understanding the impact of food, good and bad is one of the most powerful weapons we have to deal with the challenges. Our bodies are extremely clever and adaptable given the right ammunition. Science is beginning to understand that "we are our bugs" and that bacteria are the most adaptable life form on the planet … so there is hope. With our evolving knowledge of the human body we need to adapt more intelligently to the world around us.

If we do not engage, we may find that we will continue to be manipulated and unwisely served by the food and pharmaceutical industries that have our money but not necessarily our well-being in mind. All along expecting us to happily put in our mouths what they produce.

Empowerment

So clearly there is a lot more we can do for ourselves to enhance our well-being that is not necessarily being offered to us by doctors, pharmaceuticals, policy makers, public authorities, institutions, big business, marketing men and the media.

We need to ask more pertinent questions about our own on-going health. We need to simplify our daily lives and reject many 'products' we do not need. The money we save could go towards better quality, well produced food.

Reclaiming Lost Wisdom

Not only our food but our habits and attitudes need to be reassessed. One of the reasons family is so important is for the continuity of basic knowledge that can be passed down the generations. There is much wisdom that is being lost as the modern world, in all its rush and excitement, is fragmenting and veering off course.

Giving our body the nutritional help it needs significantly enhances our ability to repair. Indeed if we feed ourselves properly we can exit the fog created by poor lifestyle and have the energy and clarity to achieve a whole lot more.

CHAPTER 2:   EXPOSING OUR MISTAKES

Overfed And Starving – How Did We Manage It?
Many of us are constantly consuming whilst failing to feed our bodies.
- We are surrounded by food that is advertised as 'healthy' but isn't.
- We are surrounded by the constant temptation of junk food.
- For all the money that is spent on processed food, it does not serve us well.
- Processed food is generally nutrient poor, high in sugar and low in fibre.
- Processed food can be so tampered with that our body no longer recognises it as food or knows what to do with it.
- We are living in a complex and profit driven world where finding and preparing fresh, wholesome food is increasingly difficult.
- The way we eat today slows down our physical and mental agility.
- We feel we do not have the time or energy to prepare food from scratch.

It's a vicious circle

… And to those out there that have been dieting for decades there has to be a reversal of mind set from:

Food is bad   "it makes me fat"
To
Food is good   "it makes me healthy, energetic and protects me from disease"

The Age Of Convenience
The expression "we want to have our cake and eat it too" is possibly appropriate for western society.

As mentioned previously we have signed up for all the products of convenience. Fast food when we are out and about, pre-prepared meals when at home. An army of sprays and chemicals to make cleaning super easy. An array of grooming products to allow us to keep going for 24 hours plus, without washing! We have an expectation of jetting off on sunny holidays. We want the latest gadgets. We work our socks off to buy all these things.

The Adverts Show Us How We Can Do This

For even though we started our day tired, after a bad night's sleep reading our tablet for too long or watching telly too late … Even though we had a fairly mediocre lunch that has not given us much nutritional sustenance … Even though towards the end of the day we have a splitting headache… Even though we have a social get together over drinks this evening and we really do not feel great …. We know that it doesn't matter, we can just keep going because the marketing men have told us that the pharmaceutical guys are thinking about us. They've got this great medication that you can pop into your mouth that will give you "targeted" and "fast-action" "relief". So you can slip the pack of magic back into your pocket, tap it with appreciation and stride off confident that you can now manage an evening of …. Indulgence.

Over Medicated

Western society literally chomps its way through a mountain of medication: aspirin, ibuprophen, steroids, paracetamol, antacids, statins, painkillers, antidepressants, antibiotics, etc, that can leave us, often, with more problems than we set out with.

We run faster and faster in ever decreasing circles, created by modern living. Instead of trying to take back control, we succumb to the following:
- Stress
- Indulging in the wrong foods
- Lack of sleep and exercise.
- Our bodies try to put the brakes on with symptoms that warn us we need to slow down or change our ways.
- Our response is to go to the doctor or the chemist and seek a magic bullet in the form of medication.
- We want something that takes immediate effect.
- The medication masks our symptoms.
- We do not modify our behaviour.
- We simply carry on.
- Until the symptoms get worse and we go back to the doctor.

Sinking In A Sea Of Low Level Illness

Every time we put something in our mouths it should be something to help our bodies not leave us worse off, be it medication or food.

The quantity of sugared food, refined carbohydrates and much of the processed food we eat causes us:

Bloating	Reflux	Flatulence	Diarrhoea	Pain
Headaches	Cramps	Lethargy	Fatigue	Constipation
Increased Weight	Depression	Mental Issues	Arthritis	Heart Disease
Weakened Immunity	Cancer			

Prevention

So much of this is preventable. One day this word will become the mantra of all our doctors but there is no time to do more than patch a patient's symptom with medication. Patients need to be advised how to prevent the symptoms from happening again. Our over-worked doctors are sinking in a sea of preventable low-level illness that, unfortunately, goes on to become more serious disease.

Sleep Walkers

We have chosen to mask the symptoms of our bad habits with ever-stronger medication. Even basic paracetamol is consumed, by us and given to our children, far too readily. We have been sleep walking around the key issues that affect our health for several decades. Today there is more cause for concern for their cumulative effect.

CHAPTER 3: SUGARS OR FATS?
WHAT SHOULD OUR MAIN SOURCE OF FUEL BE?

"Your health and likely your lifespan will be determined by the proportion of fat versus sugar you burn over a lifetime ...." **Dr Ron Rosedale** MD
Dr Ron Rosedale Specialist in Nutritional & Metabolic Medicine Northwestern University Medical School USA

Our Ancestors Wouldn't Have Survived If Skipping Breakfast Made Them Wobbly
In today's society we have become predominantly sugar burners, every day, all year round. Yet we evolved to be predominantly fat burners; factoring in a cycle of sugar burning regularly but *far* less frequently.

Mother Nature Compelled Us to Seek Sweetness
In the Northern Hemisphere our early hunter, gatherer ancestors would have been on the move, with no access to stored food. Their frequency of eating compared to our constant access to refrigerators full of food highlights a huge difference in their and our feeding patterns. In addition, they had a limited seasonal opportunity to indulge in fruits. Nature provided them with seasonal berries at the end of the summer whose sweetness would compel them to eat in abundance and enable them to rapidly deposit body fat to help them through the cold, winter months.

Switching Fuel Sources with Ease
The organs, fat and muscle of a hunted animal would have been consumed in that order of nutritional preference by our ancestors. Meat and fish would have been consumed alongside tubers and plant foods, for example, offering resistant starch to feed the healthy bugs in the gut. Yet their bodies would have been well adapted to burning fat and sugars enabling them to switch back and forth with ease.

Our ancestors would have never survived from one hunt to the next if we are to believe that breakfast is the most important meal; that you *must* have three meals a day to keep your blood sugars stable! Instead, primed to use fat for fuel they were physically agile and mentally alert, ever ready to hunt down their next meal. As fat burners, they were *unlikely* to hit a "wall" mid hunt and have to resort to glucose tablets, a sport drink or chocolate!

Skipping Breakfast

For many of us today, used to permanently burning sugars – running out sends us cold turkey and makes us feel awful – leading us to rush for another fix of carbohydrate. If you feel you cannot skip breakfast, ultimately this is not a good sign, as it highlights that the body does not have the enzymes or correct hormone signalling in place to easily switch from burning sugar to fat. This is known as being metabolically flexible or 'fat adapted'.

Burning fat for fuel allows the body to enter a state of repair and to produce ketones, enhancing mental performance. **Fat can be viewed as a clean fuel,** as long as the source of dietary fat is of good quality such as quality olive oil or animal fat from healthy, antibiotic-free, pasture fed animals. Grain fed animals will have higher levels of pro-inflammatory omega 6 in their fat. [1] See Chapter 8.

Burning sugar for fuel causes oxidation and this speeds up the ageing process. For this reason **sugar can be viewed as a dirty fuel.**

If we primarily use sugar/glucose for fuel
-       We are much more likely to suffer brain fog and lethargy
-       It sends us down a path toward bowel and gastric issues, inflammatory conditions, autoimmune disorders, heart disease, strokes and cancer.

If we primarily use fat for fuel
-       We perform noticeably better both mentally and physically and for longer.[1a]
-       Endurance athletes who burn fat for fuel instead of "carb-loading" are at an advantage because sugar storage capacity in the body is limited, whereas a person may have access to 20-40,000 stored calories in their body fat.

A Better Understanding of How to Prevent Dementia

A lifetime of burning too much sugar over fat is considered to be one of the primary reasons for our cognitive decline in later life. Addressing this fact sooner rather than later may help many more people be less forgetful in old age. Neurons in parts of the brain of those with mild cognitive decline or Alzheimers have been shown to no longer be able to take up glucose for energy. Until recently it was believed that these neurons were damaged and no more could be done. However, recent experiments show that this is not the case. When given access to an alternative fuel source to glucose, the neurons that were thought to be defunct sprang back to life and worked better than ever. [1b] What was this alternative fuel source? *Ketones.*

What Are Ketones?

A Ketone is an organic compound, a by-product of the body burning fat. It is a fuel that favourably affects many markers of health and can reduce the prospect of heart disease. (2) Overall, your metabolism runs more efficiently on fat, producing fewer free radicals and therefore less oxidative stress that leads to ageing. Ketones are produced only when most of the sugar stored in our liver (known as glycogen) is used up. Only then, can our body access its stored fat, to fuel itself.

As less carbohydrate is coming into the body the brain will spare any available glucose in preference to the ketones that are being produced due to the body's fat burning state (known as *ketosis)*.

Ketosis – Good for the Body, Good for the Brain

The state of Ketosis is the term used to identify when our bodies burn fat for fuel, whether it be body fat or dietary fat. The word Ketosis may be a new word to many but the process that it describes is not. We should be in ketosis on a regular basis as this will slow down our ageing process.

Is Intermittent Fasting And A Higher Fat , Low Carb Diet The Way Forward?

Many communities around the world, and in the past, would not have access to so much sugar or be in the habit of grazing on snacks all day. They would have been in a state of ketosis. Today, however, many people, especially in the US have to almost take a lone stand to achieve ketosis whilst living in our western society. It can be hard to achieve with so much emphasis on fast food, coffee shops, and the constant availability of snacks everywhere. Yet more and more people are now successfully and enthusiastically pursuing ways of eating that activate ketosis because of the health enhancing benefits it gives them. There are two ways to achieve this but generally success is greater when both methods are combined:

- **Intermittent Fasting**
- **The Ketogenic Diet (higher fat, low carbohydrate)**

A Powerful Tool To Reduce Cravings

For many, intermittent fasting is a less challenging way to reduce addiction to sugar and carbohydrates. Fasting helps to reduce cravings because it is the most rapid way to rebalance insulin and the hormones that promote hunger.

The Benefits Are Too Good to Turn Back

Yet there seems to be a natural transition from intermittent fasting to the ketogenic way of eating. For fasting helps to significantly remove cravings for sugar, and refined carbohydrates such as bread and pasta. A new sense of well-being is achieved through fasting; those who adopt it find that well-being is disrupted by nutrient poor carbohydrates. Bloating, lethargy and reduction in mental clarity can return. These symptoms do not occur when eating nutrient dense foods such as vegetables, moderate amounts of fish and meat, combined with quality fats.

Have You Heard the Term 'Net Carbs'?

'Net' carbs simply means grammes of carbohydrate minus grammes of fibre, let me explain …. Consuming carbohydrates such as bread, pasta, rice, increases your sugar intake in the form of glucose. Regularly consumed, these foods push us into a state of sugar burning and keep us there.

For those who are committed to a higher fat, low carbohydrate diet and looking to enter a state of Ketosis (using dietary or stored fat for fuel) the recommendation is to limit your carbohydrate intake to between <u>20-50g per day of **'net'** carbohydrates</u>, depending on who you are. This simply means taking the carbohydrate weight in grammes and subtracting from it the weight of fibre in grammes within the food.

So, for example, 180.0g portion of asparagus will contain approximately, only 3.24g of "net carbohydrates". Carbs minus fibre content = "net carbs".

180g of asparagus =   **7.02g** total carbs

                                 <u>**-3.78g**</u> minus fibre

                                 3.24g "net carb"

If your daily target of "net carbs" is between 20-50g, you can see that there is plenty of scope to eat lots of vegetables. However, just *one half* of a bread bun used for a burger, for example, comes in at 20g and could therefore equate to nearly a whole day's quota of carbohydrate.

Feasting on Family Days

Like in all things moderation should prevail. No one should be in a permanent state of ketosis as it can counteract the benefits. So a regular "feasting" day is factored in where net carbohydrate intake is raised to between 100-150g.(3) On these days intake of dietary fat would be lowered. This is to ensure that the routine encompasses a cyclical time period where sugar is being burned by the body.

Feasting days should be less busy days as a drop in mental and physical energy will be noticeable after eating, for those who are used to being in ketosis. The ketogenic diet, as it is known, is proving to have very beneficial effects on the people who adopt it, as indicated by their health markers, including blood pressure, levels of HDL cholesterol, inflammatory markers and of course blood sugar levels. It also enables speedy reversal of insulin resistance.

Ketosis is a Normal, Healthy and an Important Process

Ketosis is often confused with the word Ketoacidosis. The confusion needs to be addressed. Unlike Ketosis, Ketoacidosis is a process that is out of control. Type 1 diabetics are at risk of Ketoacidosis because they cannot produce insulin. If insulin is unavailable blood sugars can go up dangerously high. Excessive ketones are produced causing thirst and frequent urination that can lead to loss of too many essential electrolytes such as magnesium, potassium, sodium etc. Ketosis, on the other hand, is a controlled process because insulin is available to maintain healthy blood sugar levels and a much smaller number of ketones are produced.

Ketosis is a normal, healthy process
Ketoacidosis is an unhealthy and uncontrolled process

Are You "Fat Adapted"?
Easily Switching From Burning Sugar to Burning Fat for Fuel

There is an expression you may have heard "fat adapted" or "keto-adapted". This is simply a term that describes whether the body is adapted to quickly switching from burning sugar for energy, to fat for fuel instead. Certain enzymes need to establish themselves and, if hormones such as insulin, ghrelin and leptin are out of balance it will make adaptation hard. (see page 93) Those not adapted to burning fat will:

1. Find that after 4-6 hours of not eating they will feel hungry and increasingly irritable or develop a headache.
2. Find the desire to snack between meals is overwhelming.
3. Find that a sensation of fullness after a meal is hard to achieve.
4. Find that no meal can be concluded without something sweet.
5. Find that they crave high carbohydrate foods like sugar, bread, pasta, rice.

The speed at which we are able to transition to burning fat depends on our insulin status - how often and how much insulin we have in our blood.

The fastest route to fat adaptation is a combination of:
- Fasting, during which time no insulin is released - (remember insulin is the 'fat *storage*' hormone and we want to burn fat) and
- A diet of low insulin stimulating foods. (See page 47)

The 5 Signs that Show You Have Become "Fat Adapted"
1. More energy
2. Better sleep
3. No cravings for sugar or carbohydrates
4. Greater physical endurance
5. Less hunger – pangs will subside and disappear
6. Better levels of concentration

What Are Mother Nature's Priorities?
Nature gave us sweet receptors to cause us to gravitate towards sugar. This helped us to ensure short-term survival for our primal ancestors. As we know, the fructose in fruit and sugar helped us lay on fat quickly, see us through the cold winters and increase our cellular reproduction to secure growth and reproduction. Yet Mother Nature has never been particularly concerned about good health into extended old age. As far as She is concerned once we have reproduced and raised our off spring we are of little consequence …..

Dying is Thoroughly Inconvenient!
We, as the stubborn and clever humans that we are, have different ideas to Mother Nature on the subject of health and longevity and so the elixir of life has always been

an elusive but constant goal. So the fact that we have a sweet tooth needs to be examined. It is a powerful driver that pushes us towards cellular reproduction. This is a good thing when we are growing and in the reproductive phase of our life. Yet, as we grow older and our cells are prone to contain genetic damage we should be more concerned that our cells are more frequently in a state of repair not duplication. This is only achieved when we are *not* burning sugar. As we grow older and our chances of cancer increase, being in a state of constant sugar burning will put us at higher risk of duplicating and fuelling our cancer cells to a point where medical intervention may be necessary.

Sugar Seeking Cancer Tests
It is worth noting '**how**' PET scans, used for finding cancer in patients, work. Cancerous cells thrive on sugar so the test is designed to seek out high glucose clusters. If we are in fat burning mode the duplication of our cells is minimised and the body is more focused on repair. In addition, unlike healthy cells that use oxygen to respire for energy and can use both sugar and fat, *cancer cells acquire their energy through fermentation, fuelled primarily by sugar.*

Questioning the Starting Point of All Our Cancer Research
For research, on the topic of cancer and the dangers of sugar over fat fuelling our body, I recommend Dr Thomas Seyfried, author of the epic tome "Cancer as a Metabolic Disease: On the Origin, Management and Prevention of Cancer". His lectures and interviews feature in many YouTube videos which may be a good first port of call as his epic tome retails at a mere £105.00! Yet this book is a milestone and possibly one day will be seen as a turning point for cancer research.

Is Cancer an Issue of Fuel or Genes?
Seyfried's challenge is that cancer has been viewed over-simplistically as being of genetic origin, whereas it should be viewed instead as a disease of metabolic origin. In other words fuelling our bodies with sugars is in part the trigger but also the main driver of cancer whilst the genetic element is the secondary pathway and will characterise which type of cancer occurs but is not the cause.

If This Is True, Then It Is Very Empowering To Us

Chemo and a Can of Coke?

Unfortunately cancer research seems to have nearly all its eggs in one basket, focusing its research on genetics. The metabolic element ignored to the point that many oncologists do not even warn patients to avoid sugar and carbohydrates.

Dr Thomas Seyfried's work is based in part on the work of the Nobel Laureate Dr Otto Warburg. He stated that a cancer cell is a cell that switches from oxygen for respiration as the source of energy to sugar for fermentation. Whilst healthy cells can use both sources for energy, cancer cells need sugar to survive. In his words:

"Cancer, above all other diseases, has countless secondary causes. But, even for cancer, there is only one prime cause. Summarized in a few words, the prime cause of cancer is the replacement of the respiration of oxygen in normal body cells by a fermentation of sugar".

Later in his life, Warburg believed prolonged exposure to pollutants led to the dysfunction of cells leading them to become cancerous, switching their energy mechanism from respiration to fermentation which requires sugar as fuel. Thus our sugar burning lifestyle is ideal for driving increasing rates of cancer.

Fasting can be an effective cancer prevention strategy as it stimulates the repair of cells that may have become dysfunctional due to exposure to toxins. Thus regular fasting can sweep out potentially cancerous cells before they take hold.

See Chapter 5 "Our Fear of Fasting".

CHAPTER 4: TOO MUCH INSULIN: A SPEEDY PATH TO AGEING AND DEMENTIA

We Must Get Our Heads Around Insulin
Before We Can't Get Our Heads Around Anything At All!

Don't Bore Me With The Details …..

When we understand why something is good or bad for us, we are more likely to add it or take it away from our routine. Understanding how too much insulin affects us is possibly one of the most life changing pieces of information we can address. So, please, please let me bore you with the details. I promise you it will be worth it.

No Apologies For Repetition

This part of the book is important; I make no apology if it appears that I convey the same point more than once. I want to put the information across in every which way I can in order to ensure that the concept is clear. The role of insulin, hyperinsulinemia, leading to insulin resistance has caused a lot of confusion that has lead to a much suffering. Again, however, do not take my word for it, follow up with your own research. I believe that the positive patient outcome and general improvement in both physical and mental agility in people who follow this understanding of insulin resistance, how to prevent it or reverse it, speaks for itself.

Mass Distraction?

Some now say that cholesterol has been a major distraction. (2) It is not the enemy we think it is; that we must re-educate ourselves to recognise that it is vital for longevity and that the perception we have of it is not accurate. Scientists are realising that the cholesterol issue is not about quantity, but about quality. See Chapter 9.

More importantly, perhaps cholesterol has distracted us from a far more vital health marker - our insulin status. Or in other words how much insulin we release to deal with the sugar in a slice of cake, for example?

The answer to that question is that many of us are producing too much insulin to deal with a slice of cake and it is making us ill. We need to understand why.

It's Not Rocket Science, We Can All Understand

Until we all become more aware of insulin in our daily lives we may well continue to exist in a western society that is seeing chronic disease, mental decline and diabetes affect the vast majority of the population in all age groups. Not to mention the burden that healthcare has become to our economies.

What Is Insulin?

Half a Billion Years of Evolution – It Deserves Our Attention

Insulin is the hormone that has enabled us to store fat for when food was scarce. It helps build muscle and increases cell proliferation (cell duplication). It is responsible for controlling blood glucose. How much circulating insulin we have in our bloodstream will determine the length of our life, our overall health and whether we are permanent sugar burners, or whether we can easily alternate between burning fat, or sugar for fuel.

Possibly the Best Marker for Assessing Health and Lifespan

The body is complex and there are many things that can go wrong. Hyperinsulinemia (too much insulin) would appear to be playing, however, a disproportionately big role in the West's levels of debilitating illnesses, weight gain and poor quality of life. What is staggering is the extent of our lack of understanding of insulin, our master hormone. In fact it may turn out that testing for insulin resistance through a test known as the **glucose/insulin tolerance test**, could prove to be the best blood marker for health and lifespan that you can have.

Unlucky Timing in Science?

Is it the case that we have been confounded all this time due to the fact that, historically, we were able to test blood sugar levels and cholesterol in the blood, years before we discovered how to measure insulin? As a consequence, type 2 diabetes became viewed as a disorder of blood sugar and treated accordingly, whilst in fact the blood sugar dysfunction was merely a late stage symptom of insulin resistance. This seemingly minor confusion, it could be said, has had catastrophic consequences on the health of millions of people. It has led to doctors treating a problem of too much insulin with…. more insulin.

Challenging How Type 2 Diabetes Is Perceived
Can It Be Diagnosed Years Earlier?
Do Many, Many More People Have It But
Are Simply Undiagnosed?

- A body overloaded with sugar is initially disguised by the body producing more insulin to deal with high sugar intake.
- The body can mask high sugar intake in this way for years.
- Thus avoiding the organ damage that high blood sugar levels can cause.
- We 'appear healthy' because our blood sugars 'appear healthy' due to an over production of insulin.

But A Body Overloaded With Insulin Becomes A Sick Body

- A body overloaded with insulin becomes desensitised to insulin.
- A body desensitised to insulin needs to produce more insulin to ensure that stable blood sugars are maintained.

An Insulin Resistant Body Is Less Sensitive To Insulin And Cannot Benefit Properly From Its Important Functions

- Hyperinsulinemia drives fat storage.
- Fat storage drives inflammation and insulin resistance.
- Inflammation drives disease including heart disease, strokes and dementia.
- But we don't know if our body is producing too much insulin to deal with our sugar 'habit' because

We never test for it
We are not aware of it as a population and
We are not taught how to control it through food

Years of Undetected Damage

If we did test for Insulin Resistance we would see that high sugar intake was starting a damaging process to our health *years* before we can identify it through testing our blood sugar levels. Years of undiagnosed damage can be taking place in your arteries but it is only once the body starts to become so resistant to insulin, to the point that it can lead to a dangerous level of glucose in the blood, that danger is flagged up. At this stage, one is about to enter or is entering a state of full-blown type 2 diabetes that needs to be dealt with immediately. We turn to medication to prevent damage to organs caused by hyper-glycaemia (high blood sugars).

If Type 2 Diabetes Was Viewed As Insulin Resistance;
- We would catch the condition earlier
- Treat type 2 diabetes differently and
- Not prescribe more insulin that only serves to make the condition worse.

Fortunately many now understand that Insulin Resistance can be treated. **Unfortunately** for the pharmaceutical industry the treatment is completely free – no medication or gadgets required. We can prevent and treat the condition by eating in a way that requires the production of less insulin and guarding against triggers of insulin such as stress and lack of sleep.

So, there is **nothing to sell** and therefore no money involved and this goes a long way to explaining why **the message is not getting through**. With the right way of eating, years of insulin resistance can be resolved in a matter of weeks as we allow our body to re-sensitise itself to this vital hormone.

Fat Or Thin, Most Of Us Are Insulin Resistant To Some Degree And This Will Define The Speed At Which We Age And Our Risk Of Dementia.

The Father of the Glucose/Insulin Test
Dr Joseph Kraft (author of "Diabetes Epidemic and You: Should Everyone Be Tested?") was the father of the glucose/insulin test, developed in the early 1970s. Kraft predicted, based on a US study that carried out his insulin test on 14,000 patients, that the true figure for pre-diabetic numbers in America was more likely to be two thirds of people, 65% of the population and not 33% as predicted by simply measuring blood sugars!

Is it Easy to Test For Insulin Resistance?

Dr Kraft's test for measuring insulin resistance is the most accurate test available but, unfortunately, it is not the most practical. The test involves taking 75g of glucose orally and then having a blood test once an hour for 5 hours to measure how much insulin is produced to process the glucose and how long your body takes to clear the insulin from the blood stream. This makes it a costly hospital based test. Plainly, a five-hour blood test is not practical to administer to the population at large on a semi-regular basis. There is an alternative, more practical, but less accurate version called the two-hour glucose tolerance test that takes just one blood test two hours after consuming 75g of glucose in solution. This will be a sufficiently large window to show whether there is a problem brewing.

How Does Your Body Cope with Cake?
Healthy versus Unhealthy

The five hour test, when plotted on a graph, shows quite accurately the state of health of an individual. The difference between insulin resistance and good insulin sensitivity would look like this:

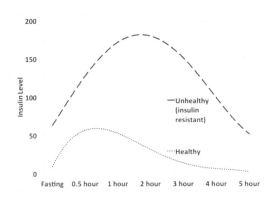

Those that require low levels of insulin to achieve normal blood sugars after eating a slice of cake are significantly healthier than those that require higher levels of insulin to achieve normal blood sugars after eating an equal amount of cake. In addition insulin will clear faster from the blood stream in a healthy person but linger longer in an unhealthy person. As long as insulin is present in the blood, any type of food consumed will be stored in the body as fat.

Signs That Tell Us Whether We Have Insulin Resistance

As a glucose/insulin test may not be easily available to many we need to recognise the signs that tell us what our insulin status may be.

As insulin's nickname is the fat storage hormone it would seem logical that the signs that indicate whether you are insulin resistant are the same as the signs that show whether you are "fat adapted".

	Insulin Resistant	Insulin Sensitive
Hungry	Yes	No
Irritable	Yes	No
Cravings for carbs	Yes	No
Lethargy	Yes	No
Anxiety	Yes	No
High blood pressure	Yes	No
Calmness	No	Yes
Energy	No	Yes
Good sleep	No	Yes
Well-defined waist	No	Yes

Waiting for Type 2 Diabetes or 'Pre-Diabetes' To Be Diagnosed Can Be Like Playing Russian Roulette

Kraft believed that insulin resistance and not cholesterol is at the core of heart disease. He theorised that everyone who died from a heart attack would have been insulin resistant for a while and on their way to type 2 diabetes; they just had not been diagnosed.

More Strokes in Younger People[1]

In many cases strokes or heart attacks are unexpected and occurring in younger and younger people. In these episodes high insulin may well have been driving on-going, undetected, inflammatory damage in the arteries. Yet high insulin levels would have, at the same time, still managed to push enough glucose into the cells to disguise and delay diagnosis of type 2 diabetes.

Just to Be Clear

In type 1 diabetes the pancreas is unable to produce insulin.

In type 2 diabetes, years of over stimulation of insulin, leads to it becoming less efficient and this is known as insulin resistance.

How to Live to Be 100?

Remember there are two common characteristics found in people who live over 100 years of age. One is high cholesterol and second is a low insulin status.

As high insulin can lead to inflammatory tissue damage (such as in the arteries) and cholesterol is produced by the body to meet the need to repair this damage then it makes sense that people who live to a ripe old age are the ones who have maintained a low insulin status. Importantly, they will probably not have been hindered by doctors trying to bring down cholesterol levels with statins.

In simple terms, tissue damage increases with age and the body will respond by creating more cholesterol to deal with repair. However, medicine has defined an arbitrary bar above which we are told cholesterol should not go. This does not in any way address the fact that the body's cholesterol production will fluctuate in response to episodes of acute or chronic inflammation taking place within the body.

Being 'Insulin Savvy' Is a Huge Advantage

Scientists and a large section of the medical community now believe that being aware of our insulin status will allow us to achieve and maintain healthy weight. It will reduce our chances of illness and mental decline significantly, yet the old views are so hard to shift, no matter how much suffering there is.

The moral of the story seems to be, if you've got a sweet tooth, regularly eat bread, pasta, rice and think you are getting away with it … chances are …. you're not!

TOFIs

It is worth noting that we have differing dispositions to how we store our body fat, depending on our genes. In simple terms there are three types of fat storage:

1.	Pear shaped – perhaps the safest of the three, where fat is stored mainly on the thighs.

2.   Apple shaped – not a good prospect for on-going health where thighs are thin but there is no visible waistline indicating that fat is being dangerously stored around the organs. Then there are the

3.   TOFIs (Thin on the Outside, Fat on the Inside) A thin person with a high body fat ratio may be collecting dangerous visceral fat around the organs whilst maintaining a thin outward appearance.

Curiously, we are seeing that you do not have to be obese to be insulin resistant and you will not necessarily be insulin resistant if you are obese, depending on your genetic disposition to certain types of fat cells. For the latest cutting edge research on the different types of fat cells and their characteristics, the Hungarian molecular biologist Gabor Erdosi is worth investigating.

Insulin is called the fat storage hormone because we cannot access and burn our body fat stores with insulin present in the bloodstream

Keeping Blood Insulin Low Makes Weight Loss Easy
The problem is that we are snacking on sugar and carbs all the time so insulin remains *ever present in the blood and takes longer to clear*. Insulin remains in the blood for 6-24 hours after eating, depending on your level of resistance, busily stacking, as fat, any carbohydrate that is being eaten. Snacking between meals, maintains high levels of insulin in the blood all the time. Losing weight becomes harder and harder as the perpetual, high levels of insulin make it impossible to access body fat stores. This is why it is far harder and slower for an individual to lose weight through calorie counting than it is through intermittent fasting, especially if the calorie counters are eating carbohydrate "a little and often". When you don't eat, you don't trigger insulin. Avoiding food for a few hours before and after a night's sleep is the easiest way to create an extended window of 'no insulin stimulation'.

Obesity is an Imbalance of Hormones Not One of Calories
Not addressing insulin not only slows down the weight loss process. It also makes an individual more prone to failure to lose weight as not addressing insulin means not rebalancing hunger and satiety hormones, leading to cravings and a desire to over eat. All this prolongs the body's unhealthy state.

How To Control Insulin In Our Body

Knowledge is power …. Understanding what triggers insulin and knowing how to prevent over-stimulating insulin could well be the difference between:

HEALTH vs ILLNESS - VITALITY vs LETHARGY - LUCIDITY vs DEMENTIA

To Control Insulin We Need to Cut Down on the Carbs *Not* the Healthy Fats

1. Fat and Protein are the only dietary sources of material for the building blocks in our body.
2. Carbohydrates provide energy but are not used by the body to build and repair.
3. **Insulin is released by:**
   a. *Carbohydrates most significantly*, **especially sugar, refined and low fibre, grain based food.**
   b. *Protein much less so.*
   c. *Fat negligible.*

4. Caloric Energy in:
   a. Fat is 9 calories per gramme of energy
   b. Protein is 4 calories per gramme of energy
   c. Carbohydrate is 4 calories per gramme of energy

This is important because if you take out energy rich carbohydrates from your diet you need to replace that energy with energy rich fats.

5. Let's Take An Example of 50g of Asparagus (4 spears) and
                               50g of White Flour (1 bread bun)

6. The Energy Difference Between High and Low Fibre Carbohydrate:
   a. 50g of asparagus contains 12 calories of energy whilst
   b. 50g of white flour contains 182 calories of energy

7. The Difference in Net Carb Value Between asparagus and white flour is revealing:
   a. 50g of asparagus contains 1.1g of net carbohydrate whilst
   b. 50g of white flour contains 37g of net carbohydrate.

Why Is This Information Important?
(This is Especially Relevant to People Who Do Not Wish to Lose Weight)
The above information is important because we have to understand that if we remove high energy food like bread, pasta, rice, etc we have to replace it with high energy fats, if we are not aiming to lose any more weight.

Let's recap on what we know:
- Between 25-50g of Net Carbs per day, depending on the individual should keep you in fat burning mode. This can still represent nearly half a kilo of fibre-rich vegetables!
- But if you look at point 7. you will see that the equivalent of just one, white flour bun will consume almost your entire carbohydrate quota for a day if you wish to stay in ketosis.
- Because the carbohydrate content is so low in vegetables and is buffered by fibre, your body does not need to release much insulin, and in this situation the dietary fat you consume will be accessible for fuelling your body instead of sending it off to be stored as fat.

So What Does a Nutrient Rich But Insulin Sparing Meal Look Like?
Just because it is suggested that an insulin sparing approach to food means eating a low carbohydrate, higher fat diet, doesn't mean that fat and protein will dominate the space on your plate. Staying within 25-50g of net carbs in a day allows for plenty of vegetables. As vegetables are quite low in calories and therefore energy, an increase in fat is needed to meet the shortfall created by removing grain-based foods. Those that are overweight do lose their weight quite quickly but once the body finds homeostasis (happy balance) you are unlikely to become underweight as long as you are eating nutritiously and increase your healthy fats.

Our plates should be abundantly filled with a varied selection of colourful vegetables, in particular green ones. Fattier cuts of meat or fish should be a small feature on the side of the plate (deck of cards in size) and a much more liberal portion of healthy quality fats should also feature, including olive oil, butter from pasture fed cows, avocadoes, nuts and seeds, cheese, coconut oil and eggs.

Increased *healthy fats in the diet will increase health*. They will also increase satiety, giving a truly lengthy feeling of fullness, provide and enable the absorption of fat soluble vitamins A, D, E and K and raise so called good cholesterol (HDL).

Apart From Sugars and Low Fibre Carbs,
What Else Must We Avoid That Triggers Insulin?
Stress has a significant affect on insulin production, as such it must be managed through exercise and forms of meditation or hobbies that distract us from our worries.

Lack of Sleep – sleep should ideally be a good quality 7 hours. Not getting enough sleep has a significant effect on insulin production. Stress and lack of sleep releases cortisol (our stress hormone). Cortisol disrupts our insulin signalling, leading to more insulin resistance as well as an imbalance of our hunger hormones. *A bad night's sleep could well lead to poor food choices the next day.*

Frequency Of Eating – Remember, the more often you eat the more frequently insulin is released and the more time the body spends with insulin in the system. When you do eat, consume nutritious food and eat until you have reached satiety.

Many People Have Two Fundamental Fears That Must Be Addressed If They Want To Successfully Control Insulin

Our Fear Of Fat And Our Fear Of Fasting

CHAPTER 5:   OUR FEAR OF FASTING

People's Success In Intermittent Fasting Has Seen Its Popularity Grow
Sufficient people in the west have now taken up the age-old intervention of intermittent fasting and are demonstrating its remarkable health benefits and power to achieve, healthy, speedy, weight loss. Knowing a little more about insulin now, you can understand why. The main benefits described in clinical reports are:

1. Improves sensitivity to insulin and leptin (see page 93)
2. Potential for slowing bone mineral density loss
3. Assists repair of DNA
4. Enhances brain function
5. Increases lifespan
6. Decreases abdominal fat
7. Decreases inflammation
8. Potential to rejuvenate the immune system
9. Reduces the risk factors that contribute to diabetes, heart disease, cancer and ageing.

A Word Of Warning
If you are diabetic, and on medication to lower blood sugar, fasting should be done under the supervision of your doctor. Bringing down blood sugar through diet or fasting while being on medication that does the same thing may bring a person's blood sugar too low and they could become *hypoglycemic.*

It must also be highlighted that intermittent fasting is not suitable for everyone especially growing children, pregnant women, mothers who are breast-feeding and type 1 diabetics. If embarking on intermittent fasting, it is even more important to eat fresh, healthy, nutritious food.

Fasting should <u>not</u> be equated with starvation. Fasting helps to re-sensitize insulin. Fasting triggers a process called autophagy that enables the body to clear out old, damaged cells. The Japanese scientist, Yoshinori Ohsumi, won the Nobel peace prize in 2016 for his work on autophagy, showing how fasting may be a very powerful cancer prevention strategy or cancer cure. See Chapter 11.

Why Calorie Counting Is Being Replaced
By A Renewed Fashion For Fasting

Counting Our Way to Failure

We have been counting calories for nearly a century now and little good it has done us. Most of us probably know someone who has been on calorie controlled diets, dedicated themselves to exercise and managed to lose a little weight or a reasonable amount of weight only to put it all back on again and then some.

Greedy and Undisciplined Failures?

It has been decades of misery and still it goes on. Many people have been made to feel like greedy, undisciplined failures. This is a totally unfair conclusion. Combatting hormones that have evolved to enable us to survive in nature but work against us in our modern world was always going to be close to impossible. Obesity is driven by an imbalance of hormones, not of calories.

Discovering our Master Switch and Weight Loss Success

If you are trying unsuccessfully to lose weight, know that insulin is like a master switch to our hunger and satiety hormones. Control the insulin, control these hormones, control the cravings. Failure to lose weight has everything to do with being fed a lot of misinformation.

Calorie counting without acknowledging insulin prevents access to an unlimited supply of energy in our fat stores that would make weight loss so much easier and successful.

Will Fasting Slow Down My Metabolism?
No

The Issue of Fast or Slow Metabolism

If we go from consuming around 2000 calories a day, for example, down to 1500 calories; after a while our body will lower its basal metabolic rate (BMR) as a survival mechanism response. This will allow the body to slow down in order to carry out all the essential body mechanisms that it needs to survive on the new anticipated intake of only 1500 calories a day. In so doing our energy levels will drop and we may not find it so easy to keep warm. In fact, our body will adapt all sorts of body processes

51

to require less energy to function. The body ends up re-adapting to the new, lower 1500 calories-a-day regime but compensates by functioning on a "go-slow".

Bigger Than Before
At this stage, our weight loss may plateau or even start to go back up again, no matter how little we seem to eat. We feel tired, grumpy, hungry and, chances are, we will return to consuming 2000 calories a day.

Unfortunately, our body views the additional 500 calories as excess, as it has readapted to 1500 calories for survival, and we are likely to put on even more weight than before.

Surprisingly, Our Metabolic Rate Can Be Increased By Fasting
By focusing on techniques and types of food that do not raise insulin instead of just reducing calories, we can manoeuvre the body towards a major advantage that many lose sight of when they worry that fasting will lower their metabolic rate….

Go On Treat Yourself to a Calorie Expending Spree!
The advantage is that, unlike with the restriction of calories to only 1500 or less, when you fast and keep your insulin levels low, you finally allow your body to tap into a *limitless* energy reserve in terms of the fat stores that you are wanting to burn off. With this limitless supply of energy your body goes on the equivalent of a spending spree, burning energy liberally, allowing you to feel vibrant and happy and not grumpy and lethargic. (1) It is no longer concerned that calories are *limited,* nor that energy must be conserved.

When to Fast and When to Feast?
This is one of the reasons why people who fast report that they feel so much more energetic than usual. In addition, they experience a heightened level of mental alertness due to the productions of ketones that are a by-product of the body burning fat. Achieving much more in a fasted state in their daily tasks, leads some to choose to fast on busy days and "feast" on family days! Realistically, this varies between people depending on their situation.

Thrive or Simply Survive?

The whole process of readdressing your insulin levels through less frequent eating patterns and, in particular, through lower carbohydrate consumption, means that you can control any previous sugar addictions. This is another reason why you will feel an increased sense of well-being. In addition, other factors kick in. For example the body uses magnesium in order to break down sugar. If the magnesium no longer needs to be side tracked to metabolising sugar it can be used instead in some of the 300 metabolic processes that allow the body to run efficiently.

For Your Own Research

For a comprehensive manual on good fasting techniques and advice, I recommend Dr Jason Fung's book called "The Complete Guide to Fasting: Heal Your Body Through Intermittent, Alternate Day and Extended Fasting", published in 2016. Fung is a Canadian kidney specialist and, as such, was receiving many type 2 diabetic patients with kidney problems in his clinic.

When he embarked on using fasting to help his patients, he was treated as a pariah by other doctors within the immediate medical community but Fung describes the results for his fasting patients as "unbelievable". As time progressed doctors around him witnessed the extensive success stories and remained impressed.

Type 2 diabetes has, until recently, been viewed as incurable. Dr Fung's type 2 diabetes patients, under his supervision, were losing weight, reducing and then coming off their medications, and experiencing vastly improved health and vitality.

Our Bodies Will Burn Available Sugar Before Being Able to Burn Stored Fat

The liver stores approximately 8 hours worth of sugar in the form of glycogen. This energy has to be used up first before we have a chance of accessing our fat stores.

Visualize A Fridge/Freezer

The best imagery I have seen to express this is found in Fung's book. He compares our liver to a fridge, used as a short-term energy/sugar store, the rest of our body tissue is compared to a deep freezer chest used as a long term energy/fat store. The fridge must always be emptied before accessing the freezer. Our problem is that we keep topping up the fridge and so the freezer contents are out of reach to us. Fasting allows the body time to burn off the sugar in the liver/fridge.

How to Ease Your Way Into Fasting

Eating dinner reasonably early, say 7pm and eating absolutely nothing else before bedtime, then sleeping for 7-8 hours will give the body, after having completed digestion, several hours fasting time. At this point sugar in the fridge will have been used up and access to the fat in the deep freezer should become available.

Depending on where one sits on the insulin spectrum will determine whether one is a grumpy, wobbly and hungry mess until breakfast. How quickly we can clear our system of insulin determines our ability to smoothly coast with ease to lunch because we have been able to tap into our fat stores.

Turn Breakfast to Brunch and Then Brunch to Lunch

Pushing breakfast later and later into the morning will increase the duration of the fast. The harder you find this to do the more important it is that you do it, but in small increments. Maybe push breakfast on by 15 minutes each day. Even if no weight is lost initially, the fasting process will immediately begin to reduce insulin circulating in your blood and start to fix your hunger and satiety hormones.

Ideally we need longer periods of time between our meals where no insulin is being released. Each one of us has to feel our own way.

Golden Rules

- Absolutely no snacking - to reduce the number of times insulin is triggered
- Eat dinner earlier and consume nothing else before bed.
- Do not eat high insulin stimulating food (sugar and grain based food)
- Replace lost energy through lower carbohydrates with a higher amount of quality fats that do not trigger insulin. See Chapter 8.
- Eat nutrient dense food.
- Avoid alcohol

Popular Timing Methods Used for Intermittent Fasting

1. Eating twice a day within a 6-8 hour window; choosing to either have breakfast and lunch or lunch and dinner. This enables a daily fast of 16-18 hours over a 24 hour period.
2. One meal a day, five days a week.
3. Alternate days fasting.

There are many different ways of fasting and a lot of studies, experience and knowledge documented on this topic, especially over the last few years, though man has practiced fasting and been aware of its benefits for thousands of years.

Dr Fung's "Complete Guide to Fasting" is an excellent resource as a first port of call, for those nervous about embarking on fasting.

Regaining Our Intuition

There are very many different formats for fasting. We all have to see what works best for us. We have to monitor how we feel, whether we are achieving benefits and making sure that we maintain a healthy focus on nutrition. We have had so many years of people telling us what to do, that we have lost our intuition and ability to listen to our bodies. When we reconnect, especially after reversing sugar addiction, many find that they are more in tune to body signals, even down to specific mineral cravings.

Warnings

1. The longer the duration of the fast, and time that the gut has remained idle, the more important it is to re-introduce easy to digest, food back into your gut. A longer fast followed by a heavy meal with fibrous vegetables, for example, has "explosive" potential.
2. Keep hydrated whilst fasting but do not over do it as
3. Salt levels need to be maintained, especially potassium, sodium and magnesium.
4. In fact sometimes a hunger sensation can be due to a lack of salt. Keeping some mineral salt with you may be useful.

What to Snack on When Not Yet Fat Adapted
You need foods that will hardly trigger insulin, are nutritious and make you feel full. The best combination to achieve this is fat and fibre, such as olives, avocados or a few nuts … or, as many people have discovered, you can try entering ….

…. The Strange World of Bullet Proof Coffee
My Neapolitan grandfather would turn in his grave if he knew that I might be advocating such a thing! It warrants mentioning because I know it has helped thousands of people succeed in the early days when they first start fasting and has enabled them to go on to succeed in their weight loss and health seeking journeys.

Bullet proof coffee is black coffee with coconut oil and, for some, butter mixed in. Personally I have never added butter but I have to admit I do quite enjoy a black espresso with a teaspoon of coconut oil. Ssshh! Don't tell the Italian relatives ….

Why Consume Such a Thing?
Coconut oil and in particular a refined version called MCT oil (medium chain triglyceride) is a flavourless oil made up of extracted Caprylic and Capric acid. These fatty acids bypass your digestive tract and go straight to the liver producing ketones, for the brain. So, MCT oil offers ketones and the mental and physical energy benefits they offer without having burned any fat. For those transitioning to 'fat adaptation', this offers a little hand up. By diminishing cravings for sugar and carbs, MCT oil helps improve insulin levels but like all things, moderation is key. When it comes to oils, I still prefer the fragrant, bountiful properties of a good quality olive oil on my food … just like my Neapolitan grandfather would have enjoyed.

NB – Too much coffee should be avoided and MCT oil should be predominantly Caprylic and Capric acid; if Lauric acid is present in any significant amount then it is a brand that is cutting corners.

Coconut Oil and Alzheimers
Currently, MCT oil or more specifically ketones available from outside the body or through diet is being studied closely in relation to helping increase cognitive function for patients with Alzheimers or in its prevention. [2,3]

Alzheimers is understood to be a disease where the brain is no longer able to obtain energy from glucose. It was believed that neurons in the brain were dying or becoming less functional causing them to become unable to utilize glucose. Recently however scientists have developed a tracer that is able to follow ketone activity in the brain and this has enabled scientists to see that, in fact, the neurons were not dying, because although their ability to utilize glucose was compromised, they became active again in the presence of ketones. This may have exciting possibilities for the on-going research in the reversal or prevention of Alzheimers.

CHAPTER 6: OUR FEAR OF FAT

Going Against the Grain

More and more studies are being published that go against the established conclusions connecting saturated fat with heart disease and the need to substitute fats for more grains to stay healthy. (1,2) In addition, replacing saturated fat with supposedly 'heart healthy' polyunsaturated fats can actually raise the risk of heart disease. Scientists researching in this area believe that the current guidelines that promote a high carbohydrate, low fat diet "should be seriously reconsidered". (2)

A study, published in The Lancet in 2017, that monitored 135,000 men and women over 7.4 years in 18 countries went as far as concluding that not only was there no association with saturated fat intake and heart disease or all cause mortality but that higher saturated fat in the diet was associated with lower risk of stroke. (4)

This last statement should perhaps be tempered with the statement that like all things the source of the saturated fat is important. Animal fat for example will only be as healthy as the food the animal has been fed in its lifetime. Grain fed animals or those given concentrate will not produce the same beta-carotene and vitamin rich, yellow coloured fat that an animal that has been pasture fed will produce. The food the animal consumes will even alter the nature of its fat from healthy saturated to polyunsaturated (less healthy when consumed in quantity and especially when heated). (5)

Fear and Misinformation Have Lead Us Away From A Vital Food Source

For the chronology of the demonization of saturated fat; a woeful story of bad science, politics and vested interest, see Chapter 8.

We need to understand the pros and cons of different types of fat, which fats to use and which to avoid and to realise that saturated fat, is our friend not our foe. Chapter 8 "Unravelling Fat" summarizes this complex topic that has been at the centre of much fear mongering and misinformation for decades. It has led us to consume unnatural and toxic vegetable oils and frightened us away from healthy animal fats, abundant in nutrients and vital fat soluble vitamins. Healthy saturated fat provides us with energy and it barely triggers insulin at all. It also raises our so-called 'good cholesterol' (HDL), an inescapable requirement for longevity.

The Fundamental Components of Our Body

It is worth remembering that the building blocks of our body come exclusively from the proteins and the fats we eat.

Our Low Fat Diets Have Made Us Bigger

The more we have swapped fat for carbohydrate the larger we have become. This will have affected not just the people who indulged in too much sugar but also those that were trying to be healthy because we were taught that eating carbohydrate, over fat …. a little and often, was better.

Burying Inconvenient Data

After years of encouraging us to fear fat in our diet and promoting a low fat, high carbohydrate way of eating the American Heart Association buried a vital statistic on page 'e81' of a 300 page report (which can be viewed online). In their 2015 report "Heart Disease and Stroke Statistics" they wrote:

"In a pooled analysis …. from 11 cohort studies in the United States, Europe, and Israel that included 344,696 participants, (the studies showed that) each 5% higher energy consumption of carbohydrate in place of saturated fat was associated with a 7% higher risk of CHD (heart disease)".

In other words the more fat we took out of our diet and the more carbohydrates we put in, the higher our risk of coronary heart disease became. You may want to read that again, and yes, this came from the American Heart Association.

Of course many know now that all those "low-fat" foods that we were told were healthy would have been better avoided. In addition taking out the fat removed the flavour and manufacturers added sugar to compensate.

A Major Caveat

The heavily promoted "healthy" polyunsaturated plant, seed and vegetable oils can be anything but healthy. This kind of fat contains high levels of pro-inflammatory Omega 6 that should be balanced with anti-inflammatory Omega 3. Instead, however, with modern diets, some are consuming 20-25 times more pro-inflammatory Omega 6 versus anti-inflammatory Omega 3, especially if consuming processed food, fast food or restaurant food (with a few exceptions). The Omega fats are also explored in more detail in Chapter 8.

Fats to Focus On
The fats to focus on are the poly-unsaturated Omega 3 fat from small, oily fish, mono-unsaturated fats like cold pressed olive oil, avocado and saturated fats like coconut oils and animal fats including butter from healthy, pasture raised animals.

Face Down, Chewing Veg for Hours ….
When we cut out the high energy/calorie carbohydrates like bread, pasta and rice to keep insulin low we cannot replace that energy with vegetables alone. We must increase our fat consumption back to what it was many decades ago, before we turned to sugar and more grains for energy, and the consequent increase in heart disease. Adding fat and a little protein to some vegetables, rich in fibre, will enable us to meet our energy requirement without having to graze like sheep … face down for hours in a plate of veg!

We Must Replace Carb Energy With Fat Energy
Lowering the amount of grains in the diet may cause an unwanted loss of caloric energy. Fat can replace that energy. View a salad, for example, as a vessel to enable you to consume a good amount of good quality olive oil, rich in phytonutrients or butter on steamed vegetables. The presence of fat will allow you to absorb the fat-soluble vitamins in your salad or greens and it will also help to leave you feeling fuller for longer.

Trying To Reverse The Established Guidelines
There are a growing number high profile professionals from all areas of the medical and scientific world that are advocating for a reversal of the dietary guidelines away from high carbohydrate, low fat toward high fat, low carbohydrate diets. UK cardiologist Dr Aseem Malhotra, often seen in the media, recently made a speech at an all-party Parliamentary session regarding diabetes in the UK, entitled "The Science of Reversing Type 2 Diabetes with a Low Carbohydrate Diet (And Overcoming Opposition from Vested Interests)".

Dr Malhotra made a very powerful speech that can be viewed on YouTube and began with a quote by Stephen Hawkins:
"The greatest enemy of knowledge is not ignorance, it is the illusion of knowledge."

All the people involved in this session are actively pursuing a reversal of our existing dietary guideline in line with the new understanding of the underlying causes of type 2 diabetes, heart disease and other chronic inflammatory diseases, relating to insulin.

One of the other contributors was Dr Zoe Harcombe, an internationally known professional who has been researching for twenty years, the subject of diets, diet advice, obesity, eating disorders and food cravings. Her perspective is 360 degrees as she was a vegetarian herself, for 20 years, but no longer. Her contribution to this Parliamentary session was extraordinary in its simplicity. Of note was:

1. The material for the building blocks of our body come from fat and protein. That is why we talk about 'essential fats' and 'essential proteins'. There are, however, no 'essential' carbohydrates.
2. As far as the macro nutrients are concerned, there exists a general consensus across the board that protein should represent approximately 15% of total calories. The argument lies in how much should be consumed of the remaining calories in the form of fat and carbohydrate.
3. Current guidelines advise that we should consume 55-60% of our total calories from carbohydrate but this means our fat intake is left at only 30%. In other words we are sacrificing an essential macro nutrient for a non essential one.
4. By advocating such a high percentage of carbohydrate we have been diverted from consuming the fat-containing animal foods that Mother Nature has packed with all the essential proteins, vitamins and minerals, because we are told too much fat will clog our arteries and kill us.
5. The decision to introduce the guideline to reduce fat intake by 30% was taken by US Senator George McGovern (a politician, not a scientist), in 1977, based on no evidence. (That evidence has still not been produced, some 42 years later). The US guideline was subsequently taken on by other governments in the west. (See page 70, The Demonisation of Fat).

6. This demonisation of fat has been embedded in our psyche for decades. So even though headlines in 2015 proclaimed that science had got it wrong and that animal fat is, in fact, healthy, in 2019, still nothing has really changed. This is also despite the fact that data continues to grow to support and confirm that dietary fat guidelines have no evidence base.(6)   In the presentation to Parliament, Dr Harcombe, referenced 17 other research papers that reached the same conclusion. These 17 papers between them had identified 40 published papers that concluded that there was no evidence, whatsoever, that showed that total or saturated fat lead to all cause mortality, coronary heart or vascular disease, strokes or heart attacks.(7) Three papers were found to the contrary but when examined closely, the data could not hold up to scrutiny.
7. Non of this research was considered by Public Health England, who, in 2016 reviewed their "Eat Well Plate" guidelines but left carbohydrate and fat recommendations unchanged.
8. Dr Harcombe studied the 2016 Eat Well Plate in detail and broke down the recommendations of the different food groups into percentages as follows:

    62%   Grain based food, including bread, pasta and rice
    8%   Vegetables and fruit
    6%   Dairy (so important for calcium and bone health)
    11%   Meat (our most important nutrient source)
    9%   Junk food!
    4%   Fats and spreads

9. It was pointed out that not only did some of the recipes, recommended in the guidelines, encourage an intake of 375g of carbohydrate in a day but also that the diet is nutritionally deficient in the following nutrients:
    - Only a quarter of our requirements of fat soluble vitamins A (in Retinol, a form vital for eye health and only available in animal foods)
    - Only a quarter of our requirements of vitamin D3 (also only available from animal food, Vitamin D2 but not D3 is available in plant foods).
    - Less than half our requirements of fat soluble vitamin E.
    - And finally, calcium.

10. Pulling no punches, Dr Harcombe begs the question, is it not surprising therefore that the reason our society is in the midst of a diabetic epidemic is simply because our bodies cannot handle all this carbohydrate in the quantities and frequency that we are encouraged to consume it in. Is it no wonder that dietary advice is a "diabetes disaster"?

11. The Public Health England panel has representatives from five associations, including the British Retail Consortium, the Food and Drink Federation, the Association of Convenience Stores, the British Nutrition Foundation and the Institute of Grocery Distribution. This last association contains the names of companies that could make your heart sink such as McDonalds, British Sugar, Mars, Kellogg's, Tate & Lyle, Pepsico, Danone, The Coca Cola Company, Starbucks Coffee, Ferrero Roche, Nestle, KP Snacks, Tesco, Unilever, Iceland, McCain, Cargill, Greggs the Bakers, Sainsbury's and Asda.

12. In conclusion Dr Harcombe politely asks the Parliamentary session to consider three things:
   - "Don't base our guidelines on the one macronutrient we do not need and diabetics cannot handle".
   - "Don't allow the fake food industry to set our guidelines".
   - "Offer patients choice. There are 3 evidence-based ways to put type 2 diabetes into remission. Patients should be offered both dietary options: low calorie *and low carbohydrate*". (Currently the options are only bariatric surgery or low calorie.)

Dr Harcombe's speech is viewable on YouTube together with the other speakers at the Parliamentary session that day.(8)

Will We See The Tables Turned on Grains As The Artery Clogging Enemy?

As we know the build up of fat (triglycerides) in the blood is dangerous but the mechanisms that create this scenario have been confused. Blame has been falsely apportioned to dietary fat, in particular saturated fat from animal sources, when in fact the true culprit has been excess carbohydrate. Or more precisely, the overload of carbohydrate energy, that we have fed our bodies.

The liver converts excess sugars from carbohydrates into fat through a process called *lipogenesis.*

So if both carbohydrate and fat end up as fat in the body why is one more problematic than the other in quantity?

The significant difference is that low fibre carbohydrates, such as sugar, flour based products, many grains and even frequent snacking on fruit, have the *ability to hinder the hormones that regulate our appetite, suppressing our feelings of fullness, driving our hunger and reducing our desire to move.* This has enabled us to over consume to a staggering degree; with more energy than we could ever hope to use up. Carbohydrate, unlike fat, triggers insulin (our fat storage hormone) which then facilitates the energy overload to be stored as fat. This can eventually lead to unsatisfactory levels of fat circulating in the blood; not able to be efficiently distributed into the cells. This can occur not only in the obese but in thin people as well.

The hormone disruption that low fibre carbohydrates, together with sugar, creates, is now seen to be a significant driving force of the chronic inflammatory diseases and cancers that we are witnessing in the west today.

Fat Is Not The Enemy.
We *must* consume higher amounts of healthy fats such as olive oil, coconut oil, butter from grass fed cows, fat and fatty meat from grass fed animals, eggs, avocadoes, nuts and seeds. Healthy fats are very nutritious especially for providing and enabling the absorption of the fat soluble vitamins A, D3, E and K. Fat and protein are the building blocks of our body and we need them for both building and repair. Carbohydrates only provide energy.

Healthy fats provide energy but *also proper satiety.* "Satiety" – definition: the condition of being full or gratified beyond the point of satisfaction; surfeit. This is not a word or a feeling that many, any longer, understand or experience. Healthy fats do not disrupt our hormones like carbs can. So we are less likely to over eat fat as we are to over eat carbohydrates.
In other words fats make you fuller faster and for longer.
This has not been properly and extensively understood until recently and
It has become a game changer in the world of nutrition.

Major Changes to Our Macro Nutrients Suddenly Popped Out of Nowhere
In the 1970s (suddenly, after thousands of years of man's existence) we were told to eat more carbohydrates, less fat. We were advised to avoid natural saturated fats and to consume the newly invented, highly processed and so-called "healthy" vegetable oils, rich in pro-inflammatory Omega 6 that is unstable, unhealthy when consumed in quantity and rendered even more unhealthy when heated. See Chapter 8.

CHAPTER **7**: INFLAMMATION = AGEING

A Word We All Need To Know More About

What's The Big Deal With Inflammation?
Understanding inflammation is an important part of learning about our health and how to achieve lasting well-being.

Is inflammation a good or bad thing?
Without inflammation, wounds and infections would never heal
But, for many, it is out of control, and at the root of a whole host of conditions.

What Is Inflammation?
It is an important part of the body's immune response and protection. It works in our bodies to remove harmful agents, damaged cells and starts the healing process. An obvious example is the puffy swollen skin around a cut, but this process goes on inside the body as well.

Know The Difference Between Acute And Chronic Inflammation
ACUTE: the body dealing with a cut to the arm is an easy example of a healthy, acute inflammatory response. The tissue surrounding the cut goes red, becomes swollen and hurts as the damaged cells release chemicals that send signals to our white blood cells to come in and clean up the wound of all damaged tissue. When done, other cells, collagen and cholesterol step in and carry out repair. Once this is done, the swelling subsides, the pain goes away, and everybody goes home!

CHRONIC: the body dealing with a constant intake of sugars, carbohydrates, crisps and fried foods as well as other toxins, viruses and bacteria or constant stress or lack of sleep. All these things lead to a perpetual state of inflammation. A response, driven by insulin, that can never subside for the attack is on-going.

This chronic cycle of repair, more inflammation, break up of repaired tissue and more repair on top of repair, is the basis of atherosclerosis (otherwise known as the hardening of, or the obstruction of the arteries). This narrowing of vessels can lead on to high blood pressure, strokes, heart attacks, or reduced blood flow to the brain, causing mental decline. Simultaneously to this, sugar consumption can trigger a host of negative chemical reactions and feed the bad bugs and yeast in our gut that all lead to, and enhance, our chronic inflammation.

How Too Much Insulin Drives Inflammation

The inflammatory process that should be beneficial, is out of control. Long before type 2 diabetes is identified, increasing levels of insulin are leading many of us to be affected in some way by inflammation that will not subside. Our bodies are continually trying to fight off foreign substances with an inflammatory response that leads to tissue damage created by the powerful chemicals released by our immune system. Unfortunately, the presence of too much insulin disrupts our immune system's Regulatory T cells that are responsible for maintaining a balance between too little and too much inflammation in the body. (1)

So The Take-Home Is:
Control Insulin, Control Chronic Inflammation, Control Disease. (1a)

The Relationship Between Our Gut, Brain, Inflammation and Mental Health

A fascinating book called Brain Maker, published in March 2015 by Dr D Perlmutter, a neurologist and nutritionist, deals in detail with the influence of gut health in protecting our brain health. Perlmutter maintains chronic inflammation and brain degeneration are closely linked.

Consuming sugar will feed the bad bugs and yeast in our gut and add to our chronic inflammation. Gut dysfunction and inflammation are linked to depression.

With inflammation now starting to be viewed as possibly a primary risk factor for depression, neuroscience today is gravitating toward studying dietary changes rather than pharmaceutical prescriptions for treatment of depression. All these foods are indeed vital but maybe we are forgetting to focus equally on another category we need to avoid (apart from sugar) that is highly inflammatory.

Omega 6, Pro-Inflammatory, Poly-unsaturated Fat ….

CHAPTER 8:   UNRAVELLING FAT

The Omega Band Wagon
Everyone has jumped onto the 'Omega Band Wagon'. How many of us, though, know anything about it? We probably take cod liver oil, fish oil or omega supplements. What do you take? Omega 3? Omega 3 & 6 combined? Omega 3, 6 & 9? Why do we take it and how much should we actually consume?

What Are Omega Essential Fatty Acids?
These are necessary for health but mostly obtainable only through diet. In essence:
Omega 3 Acts To Reduce Inflammation
Polyunsaturated Fat
Is the only Omega that may require supplementation
Omega 6 Acts To Promote Inflammation
Polyunsaturated Fat
Both Omega 3 and 6 are vital but should be consumed in equal measure.
Omega 6 is more readily available through dietary sources than Omega 3.
Omega 6 is only required in moderate quantities for the healing process.
Omega 9 Acts To Reduce Inflammation
Monounsaturated Fat. Not an essential fat as the body can produce it. Also abundant in olive oil.

NB: Omega 3 is best from animal sources such as oily fish. Plant based Omega 3 requires processing by the body to benefit in the same way as animal sources but this process is not very efficient.

The Omega 3/Omega 6 Ratio Problem [1]
Ideally, we should consume far more equal measures of omegas. Some say a ratio of 1:4, some say 1:2. However, Western society, more than at any other time in history, is consuming on average 20 times more pro-inflammatory omega 6 than anti-inflammatory omega 3. The ratio for many has become 1:20 even 1:25.

How Are We Consuming So Much Omega 6?

In the last 150 years with the advent of industrial production of vegetable oils there has been a dramatic rise of around 10-20 times the consumption of pro-inflammatory Omega 6 through processed and fast food, with some people consuming over 25 times more Omega 6 than Omega 3. (1a) This is another major reason inflammatory diseases have reached such numbers in the West.

Omega 6: Sources to Avoid and Sources to Seek

Unhealthy: Processed foods that contain inexpensive vegetable oils, such as fries, crisps, pre-prepared foods, cakes and biscuits.

Healthy: Olive oil, avocados, 'grass-fed' butter, fresh whole nuts and seeds that not only give you enough Omega 6 but many other beneficial nutrients.

The Problem With Vegetable And Seed Oils

These oils are called PUFAs (Polyunsaturated Fatty Acids) and are:

1. Generally very high in Pro-inflammatory Omega 6.
2. Unstable when exposed to heat and light and susceptible to being turned rancid and toxic during the heat-generating production processes in pre-prepared and fried foods. This is how trans fats, trans-unsaturated fatty acids or trans fatty acids are generated. They have been shown to be consistently associated with heart disease. (2)
3. Consumed in extraordinary quantities through processed food:
   Fast food, fries, crisps, cakes, biscuits, prepared meals all topped with more of the same in lashings of sauces such as mayonnaise or tomato sauce and baked produce topped with margarine.
4. Leading to chronic inflammation and disease. (3)
5. Omega 6 enables liver damage from alcohol whereas saturated fat protects the liver from alcohol abuse.
6. Omega 6 reduces our ability to absorb Omega 3. (3a)

In nature, plant oil is wrapped up tightly in small nuts and seeds
Allowing us to only access its oils in small healthy quantities
Nature did not mean us to process these foods on a vast scale.

Suddenly, in the Mid 20th Century We Were Told to Alter Our Fat Eating Habits

Have the very substances that we have been encouraged to substitute butter and animal fat for, caused chronic inflammation, especially in the quantities consumed today? We have removed saturated fat that protected us from inflammation and replaced it with a form of fat that promotes inflammation, through the promotion of vegetable/seed oils,.

How Did We Fall Out of Love with Saturated Fat –
The Demonization Of Butter Time Line

1.   Like many things, it started in America. In 1911, the first shortening product (fat to make pastry) to be mass-produced and made entirely out of vegetable oil was introduced. This was the beginning of what has become a vastly lucrative industry where vegetable oil has replaced animal fat. Oil is to be found in most processed foods and indeed in home-cooking, as people were told to fear butter and animal fat and replace it with heat processed plant oil and margarine. (4)

2.   By the 1920s-30s, heart disease was reaching epidemic levels not seen before. Doctors were finding that this 'uncommon' disease was becoming a 'common' cause of death.

3.   By 1950, doctors had forgotten a time when heart disease was uncommon.

4.   It should be noted that the consumption of saturated fat had always been a dietary staple amongst populations all over the world but what changed was the incidence of heart disease in America.

5.   With heart disease reaching very concerning levels in the US by the 1950s scientists and government were looking for answers.

6.   Into the story enters Ancel Keys, a pathologist at the University of Minnesota. A scientist who today appears on thousands of sites across the internet. Sites that villainies him for aggressively pushing his theory called the "diet-heart hypothesis", the catalyst for our fear of butter and saturated fats. (5)

7.   Ancel Keys' theory is now, said to be based on very poor science. (6)   In essence, he was very selective with his findings, only including results that fit with his theory and discarding data that didn't fit into his hypothesis. He was, however, a very charismatic, strongly opinionated man who had good connections with influential and non-scientific individuals who accepted what

he stated to be true. His public profile had gained such momentum he even had his face on the front of Time Magazine in 1961.

8.   In the same year, based on Ancel Keys' work the American Heart Association (a self-appointed body) published guidelines for the first time advising US citizens to reduce their intake of saturated fats.

9.   By 1977, this advice became official and adopted by the US government. The rest of the western world soon followed.

10.   In 1990, McDonalds replaced animal fat to cook its fries with vegetable oil.

11.   The West has followed Keys' hypothesis for over 60 years and during that time, despite best efforts and hundreds of millions spent to prove his theories, no one has satisfactorily proved him to be correct.

12.   In the meantime, and despite adopting his recommendations, we have seen heart disease become one of the western world's major killers.

A Tribute to John Yudkin Author of "Pure, White and Deadly"

At the time of Ancel Keys notoriety a less 'charismatic' but noteworthy scientist in England by the name of John Yudkin of Christ College Cambridge who worked at Queen Elizabeth College, London, was protesting that the problem lay with sugar and not saturated fat. He was aggressively discredited by Ancel Keys and the powerful sugar industry. In 1972 he wrote a book called "Pure, White and Deadly" in America it was called "Sweet and Dangerous" and had success worldwide. The last paragraph of Chapter 1 begins 'I hope that when you have read this book I shall have convinced you that sugar is really dangerous.'

In 2009, an endocrinologist, interested in childhood obesity, by the name of Dr Robert Lustig, recorded a lecture called 'Sugar – The Bitter Truth'. This lecture has been viewed many millions of times on YouTube. In it he revealed his own independent research on sugar came to the same conclusions as Yudkin. He noted his admiration of Yudkin's work and "Pure, White and Deadly" was republished for the second time in 40 years in 2012. Dr Robert Lustig has published the book "Fat Chance: The Hidden Truth About Sugar, Obesity and Disease".

Butter is Wonderful

Butter has created so much confusion and anxiety in people in the past few decades. Let's try to dispel the fear of butter and also encourage its celebration as a valuable nutritional tool. One that most of us love to eat!

For centuries cultures around the globe have valued and celebrated butter for its health benefits, cultures whose knowledge and observation of food was passed down from generation to generation, unchanged.

Butter Offers a Perfect Tool For Bringing Vitamins and Minerals Together

Fat soluble vitamins work closely with minerals found in vegetables. Adding butter to your steamed vegetables is an easy daily dish that will bring vital nutrients together in an easily absorbable way. Butter offers fat soluble vitamins A, D, E, K and assists the absorption of important trace minerals: Chromium, Copper, Manganese, Selenium and Zinc. It cannot be underestimated how important to good health these fat soluble vitamins, from animal fats, are. Yet, removal of animal fats from our diets in recent years has not served us well. Studies of traditional, non-industrialised communities attribute low levels of disease to high intake of these vitamins, through the intake of 65% of total calories from animal foods. Since we have been made to fear animal fat for decades it is likely that society at large will find it hard to shift to a different way of thinking. Fear mongering continues today intensely motivated by environmental considerations.

…. A Note on Quality: In order to obtain the many health benefits of butter the quality of the cow's diet is vital. As previously mentioned, pasture/grass fed cows produce healthy, nutrient rich yellow/orange butter (beta-carotene from the grass). Grain fed cows will not offer the same goodness and their fat and butter is whiter and waxy. The richer the pasture the cow feeds on the more nutritious the butter. In the summer and autumn butter will be at its golden best.

…. And a Note of Caution: The Real Danger of Butter

So you have been told you can have butter after all – but what are you going to do with it? The fact is we love to pile butter onto carbs! Toast, crumpets, muffins, sandwiches, cakes, none of which are healthy.

Does Anyone Want To Hear About The Benefits Of Saturated Fats?
- Saturated fat is not the cause of our modern diseases but is an important player in body chemistry and together with protein is an essential building block.
- Saturated fat is stable to cook with compared to polyunsaturated fats (see fats comparison chart at the end of this section).
- It's good for our heart, raising our so-called good HDL cholesterol. (7)
- Saturated fats and the effect on dietary cholesterol can help prevent anxiety and mood swings and even reduces levels of anger and violence that lead to unhealthy effects of stress. (8)
- It promotes a healthy immune system. (9)
- It promotes healthy bones. (9)
- Saturated fat makes up at least 50% of the cell membranes providing their necessary stiffness and integrity. (9)
- Omega-3 fatty acids are better retained in the tissues when the diet is rich in saturated fats. (9)
- Your brain needs saturated fat to fully function and in addition has the added benefit of stimulating the growth of new brain cells. (10)
- The conclusion of very many recent studies state that saturated fats are not associated with all-cause mortality, cardiovascular disease, coronary heart disease, stroke or type 2 diabetes.

What is Healthy Fat? - Which Fats/Oils To Use

Summary

Polyunsaturated Fat – Eg Vegetable and Seed Oils
- Generally high in Pro-Inflammatory Omega 6
- Contain Anti-inflammatory Omega 3
- Not stable and become toxic when cooked at high temperatures

Monounsaturated Fat – Eg Olive Oil
- Low in Pro-Inflammatory Omega 6
- Relatively stable when cooked at high temperatures
- Good quality cold-pressed olive oils contain a wealth of polyphenols and generally best consumed cold

Saturated Fat – Eg Butter, Coconut Oil, Animal Fats
- Lowest in Pro-Inflammatory Omega 6
- Stable when cooked
- Solid at room temperature

Fats Highest in Saturated Fat

Natural variation in % occur but the figures give an important understanding of the underlying ratios.

	Sat %	Mono Unsat %	Poly Unsat %	Omega 3 Anti Inflamm %	Omega 6 Pro Inflamm %
Coconut Oil	**86.5**	5.8	1.8	-	1.8
Butter	**62.0**	29.0	4.0	0.3	2.7
Palm Oil	**49.3**	37.0	9.3	0.2	9.1
Beef Tallow	**49.8**	41.8	4.0	0.6	3.1

Fats Highest in Mono Unsaturated Fat

	Sat %	**Mono Unsat %**	Poly Unsat %	Omega 3 Anti Inflamm%	Omega 6 Pro Inflamm%
Olive Oil	13.8	**73.0**	10.5	0.8	9.8
Avocado Oil	13.0	**68.0**	10.0	9.0	12.0
Rapeseed	8.0	**58.5**	29.0	5.8	23.0
Sunflower	9.0	**57.3**	29.0	-	29.0
Goose Fat	27.7	**56.7**	11.0	0.5	9.8
Duck Fat	33.2	**49.3**	12.9	1.0	11.9
Peanut Oil	16.9	**46.2**	32.0	-	32.0
Pig Lard	39.2	**45.1**	11.2	1.0	10.2
Chicken Fat	29.8	**44.7**	20.9	1.0	19.5

Fats Highest in Poly Unsaturated Fat

	Sat %	Mono Unsat %	**Poly Unsat %**	Omega 3 Anti Inflamm %	Omega 6 Pro Inflamm%
Flaxseed	9.4	20.2	**66.0**	!53.3!	12.7
Walnut Oil	9.1	22.8	**63.3**	10.4	53.0
Soybean	15.6	22.8	**57.7**	6.8	50.4
Corn Oil	12.9	27.6	**54.7**	1.2	53.5
Sesame	14.2	39.7	**41.7**	0.3	41.3

Nutritiondata.self.com

Will We Return To Cooking Our Fast Food Fries And Chips In Animal Fat? It Wouldn't Make Vegetarians Happy ... But ....

Our fries from some of the biggest fast food chains were much tastier up until the 1990s when they changed from using beef tallow to vegetable oil.

We have taken a natural, essential food like animal fat or coconut oil that has been available to man and animal for all of history, that our physiology has been built up around, and suddenly replaced it in the last 70 years with something completely different and in such enormous proportions.

The scale of industry and mass production today allows, what may seem small changes to our diet, to be magnified up into proportions that can have effects that we never anticipated and the plant oil industry may be an example of this.

Even though recent revelations have helped highlight possible dangers of vegetable oils with adverse publicity about 'trans fats' and 'hydrogenated oils' we have not tackled our disproportionately high intake of Omega 6 in plant oils.

CHAPTER **9**:   CHOLESTEROL – A Mass Distraction?

Cholesterol is Vital to Our Body and to Any Prospect of Longevity

This is a topic that is obviously a book in itself. All I wish to do here is indicate the new thinking and the new thinkers on the subject. This subject is currently being turned on its head by science. Below I have summarised as simply as possible the new picture of cholesterol that is being painted.

The Common Confusion Between Fats (Triglycerides) and Cholesterol

- The number one difference is that *fats (triglycerides) provide energy but cholesterol does not.*
- Although cholesterol and triglycerides travel together around the body cholesterol offers support, maintenance and repair to our cells but does not provide calories.
- Triglycerides offer fat energy in the form of the three fatty acids, saturated fat, mono-unsaturated fat and poly-unsaturated fat, hence the word *tri*glyceride. These fats are obtainable through the fat we eat and are also produced in our liver.
- The exceptions to this are the commonly known essential fatty acids, Omega 3 and Omega 6 that can only be obtained through diet.
- Many people confuse fats (especially saturated fat) with cholesterol, neither one can turn into the other.
- We can obtain both triglycerides and cholesterol through diet but the body also has the ability to produce both, itself.
- Dietary cholesterol, obtainable through animal foods, has little impact on how much our body produces because *we would have to eat, for example, around 14 eggs in a day to match the 3000mg of cholesterol the body makes everyday;* 1000mg in the liver and 2000mg in our cells.

Without It We Die

So vital is cholesterol that the body not only produces it but recycles it as well.

- A very small proportion of our cholesterol comes from our diet, though the body will make minor adjustments to rebalance the cholesterol it needs depending on how much we consume.

- Nearly a third of the cholesterol we produce is contained in our brain.
- It is integral to the body's immune system and
- Fundamental to the body's ability to repair tissue.
- It is the basis to the construction of nearly every cell in our body and
- Helps regulate cell signalling and neurological processes.
- It is fundamental in the production of hormones, including Vitamin D.

Lipoproteins: Fat Transporters That Carry Our Cholesterol and Triglycerides
'Lipoproteins' act as 'taxis' that allow the transport of our crucial 'fatty globules' of cholesterol and triglyceride molecules through our 'water-based' blood stream. Without these lipoprotein taxis, the fatty globules would form dangerous obstruction to the flow of blood, leading to death.   All the cholesterol in these lipoprotein taxis is the same, it is the lipoproteins that vary in characteristics and can become damaged. There are several different types of lipoproteins, the main ones to know are:

Chylomicrons:
Are lipoproteins that bring in triglycerides (fat energy for our cells) from the fat in our diet into our body. These lipoproteins carry very little cholesterol as most of it is made in the liver and does not come from our diet. So chylomicrons offer mainly fat (triglyceride) energy.

Very Low Density Lipoproteins (VLDL):
Are lipoproteins that are produced in the liver that carry triglycerides (to fuel) and cholesterol (to maintain and repair) the cells of our body. VLDLs usually stay around in the body for about 3-60 minutes. They become ….

Intermediate Low Density Lipoproteins (ILDL):
Are lipoproteins that have off loaded most of the triglycerides but still have cholesterol on board. ILDLs generally circulate in the body for about 30 minutes. They become ….

Low Density Lipoproteins (LDL):
Are lipoproteins that have off loaded the triglycerides and now just carry cholesterol. LDLs circulate for 2-3 days in the body with their "cholesterol repair/support tool kit".

They also have the ability to bind to rogue pathogens, in order to expel them from the body.

High Density Lipoprotein (HDL)

HDL cholesterol otherwise known as 'good cholesterol' does not carry triglyceride energy; it is central to protecting and maintaining healthy LDL cholesterol and taking it back to the liver for recycling. High levels of HDL are associated with good health. Saturated fat in the diet raises HDL.[1] As ever, though, the best way to maintain healthy levels of HDL is to ensure your insulin status is healthy.

An Elegant Energy Transport System

All these lipoproteins are part of an extremely elegant energy transport system[1a] carrying both cholesterol and triglycerides around our body to fuel our cells and muscles and assist in their maintenance.

What Is In LDL's Repair Tool Kit?

After off loading energy, LDL hangs around in the body with its cholesterol cargo, in order to carry out its second role in providing repair and support material, including vitamins, for cells that are in need of maintenance. In addition LDL aids the immune system by scooping up pathogens for removal from the body. Refer back to the list at the beginning of this chapter to be reminded how fundamentally important cholesterol is.

Centenarians Don't Take Statins

It is unsurprising, therefore, that cholesterol is seen in higher levels in the very old; and many studies indicate that high levels of HDL and LDL is associated with longevity.[1b] Suppressing its production through medication, the very substance centenarians have in abundance and necessary to reach such an impressive age, may be counter effective and it is arguable that statins should not be handed out just because we have elevated levels of LDL. Advanced cholesterol tests can ascertain levels of damaged LDL. This damage is strongly linked to the poor lifestyle choices that can lead to high levels of insulin, insulin resistance and glucose imbalance. Whether we are tested or not, we can all start addressing insulin resistance right away, if we think we need to.

If We Provide The Right Environment LDL Will Protect Us Well
So lingering LDL (with fat energy off loaded, but still offering immunity and repair to cells in need) can enhance our health. Yet these protective mechanisms can be disrupted if we fail to provide for our body correctly because of those infamous poor lifestyle choices.

Becoming Efficient Fat Burners Will Provide A Good Environment for LDL
As you may know, it is not good to have high levels of fat in the blood. As mentioned earlier LDL off loads triglycerides but if in the presence of too much insulin, burning of triglycerides for energy may not be efficient and we can end up with higher levels of fat circulating for too long in the bloodstream, which is not desirable. In addition HDL will try to rebalance this situation but in so doing will lead to a reduction in the body's overall HDL level that is undesirable also.

If a blood test reveals high levels of triglycerides and low levels of HDL, it is time to make changes. An increase in saturated fats will help raise HDL and a reduction in sugars, grains and low fibre carbohydrates will see a lowering in triglycerides.

Once again this highlights the importance of being aware of our insulin levels if we want LDL and HDL to do their work well and enable us to fully benefit from the "full service" lipoproteins have to offer.

Quality Not Quantity(2)
Historically the preoccupation with the so-called LDL 'bad' cholesterol has been with the **quantity** measured in our blood. Yet the results of very many studies (see page 82) show that high levels of LDL cholesterol indicate no relationship with disease, cardio vascular or otherwise. In fact, as mentioned, it is the opposite, high levels of cholesterol are associated with longevity and protection against infection and the build up of arterial plaque.(1b) In an example of many similar studies, in the American Heart Journal in 2004, heart attack patients were compared to a healthy group of people. Again and again LDL cholesterol levels across both groups showed no relevance to heart attack. Instead glucose tolerance and insulin resistance proved to be consistently, very significant.(3,4)
Yet LDL *can* become damaged (oxidised) if the body is in an inflammatory state

The Old Theory Maintained That LDL Became Damaged In Our Arteries

Over and over studies show that those with high insulin levels have more damaged LDL circulating in the blood stream and that a greater presence of sugar can bind to the proteins resulting in oxidised (damaged) LDL.(5) The traditional theory was that LDL would become damaged once it entered the arterial wall. It is important to spell out the significance of this new theory. A high carbohydrate/sugar diet can lead to oxidised LDL before the LDL particles get anywhere near the arterial wall.

What is equally important to take from this information is that a person with high levels of *undamaged* LDL can benefit from enhanced protection against infection and arterial damage, as long as *metabolic flexibility* can be maintained and we can sustain efficient fat burning.

If we eat the right foods, exercise and not overload our bodies with energy by eating more than we need, then we can protect the quality and preserve the beneficial function of LDL.

The Answer, As Always, Lies in Prevention Not 'Symptom Patch-Up'

So it would seem that the answer lies in preventing an environment that allows LDL cholesterol to become damaged in the first place. In other words taking measures to avoid hyperinsulinemia and insulin resistance, triggered by too many carbohydrates. In addition raising healthy fats in our diet raises our HDL 'good' cholesterol levels that in turn help to maintain, repair and recycle LDL and thereby help to stop it from becoming a problem.

When Sugar and Low Fibre Carbs Rear Their Ugly Heads

As usual the naughty kids on the block are sugar and low fibre carbohydrates, *although not alone*, they are a major contributor to the eventual damage of LDL. Sugar binds to the LDL protein molecules and oxidises (damages) the protein.

So What Can Cholesterol Testing Tell Us?

There is a cholesterol test that is a strong predictor of health but it is more detailed than the standard cholesterol test that most of us have. It is an advanced lipoprotein test that *measures the number of lipoprotein particles rather than the cholesterol inside the lipoproteins.* It is known as the APOB/APOA1 ratio.

APOB relates to the particles in LDL. APOA1 relates to the particles in HDL. The ratio of APOB (LDL particles) to APOA1 (HDL particles) can be a strong indication of a person's level of insulin resistance. Low HDLp and high LDLp can indicate insulin resistance and generally those that are insulin sensitive have high HDLp and low LDLp.

Current Guidelines are Counter Productive
Essentially and simplistically put, the currently recommended:
High carbohydrate intake will therefore create an environment of
raised insulin that can lead, through the inflammatory process, to more damaged LDL and
Low fat intake will lead to insufficient HDL cholesterol to manage the situation.

We Must Tackle Inflammation to Maintain Healthy LDL
If it is the *quality* of LDL not the *quantity* that counts, then the question is not how high are my levels of LDL but, are they damaged? If you are suffering from chronic inflammation then they may well be. This is why people who suffer from Rheumatoid Arthritis (a disease with chronic inflammation at its core) need to be wary of their heart health as well.

So How Do We Avoid Heart Disease?
If cholesterol is no longer a significant factor of heart disease, then what is? You guessed it ...hyperinsulinemia. Remember that by the time someone has reached the type 2 diabetic stage they have already been at much higher risk of a cardio vascular event (heart attack or stroke) for some years.

But What Else?
AVOID: - Omega 6/Omega 3 imbalance
               - Smoking
               - Stress
               - Poor sleep
               - High iron levels (ferretin). *Donating blood can help.*
SEEK OUT: - More magnesium in the diet
               - Vitamin D supplementation
               - Movement throughout the day,

- Building strength in your muscles
- Sleep - 7 hours per night and
- More high quality fats and try to
- Burn more fat than sugar
- Stress management strategies
.... And breathe ......

What the Numbers Really Show

Unfortunately we have to understand that there are very many 'experts' who are still stuck in the old dogma, preaching that high cholesterol is the cause of heart disease.

The last 50 years of official advice, telling us that saturated fat raised cholesterol and led to heart disease was based on Ancel Keys "Seven Countries Study" initiated in 1956. However further analysis of this study was carried out by Dr Malcolm Kendrick author of "The Great Cholesterol Con" published in 2008 and "Doctoring the Data" published in 2014. In his analysis Kendrick took World Health Organisation data from 200 countries. He then produced his own "Seven Countries Study" except he did two versions. One for the countries with the highest intake of saturated fat and the second version for the seven countries with the lowest intake of saturated fat. The results were consistent:

the seven countries with: **the lowest saturated fat intake had the highest rates of heart disease**

the seven countries with: **the highest saturated fat intake had the lowest rates of heart disease**

Then Dr Zoe Harcombe PhD read the work of Dr Kendrick and decided to go a step further. She embarked on analysing World Health Organisation data from 192 countries and therefore looking at results of millions of individuals worldwide to see the relationships between:

Cholesterol and death from heart disease
Cholesterol and death from all cause mortality

In all her graphs the results were the same.

The higher the cholesterol, the lower the deaths from heart disease or all cause mortality.

Dr Kendrick and Dr Harcombe have a presence on YouTube and their interviews are worth listening to. Their books and Harcombe's blog are also good sources of researched statistical data.

Track Insulin Instead of Cholesterol To Prevent Tragedy
When it comes to the nitty gritty of the mechanics of cholesterol and lipoproteins, I believe one of the men of the moment, who are throwing new light on the science, is **Ivor Cummins** author of "Eat Rich, Live Long" published in 2018. Cummins is a biochemical engineer working in the medical industry. His research of the science is showing how hyperinsulinemia is the significant driver of heart disease, not cholesterol. In addition he is putting forward intricate and compelling information on the mechanics of cholesterol or, in reality, more importantly the workings of low and high density lipoproteins. (LDL and HDL cholesterol).

"If You Don't Measure It You Can't Fix It"
Cummins seems to enjoy coming to this topic from the perspective of engineering, maintaining that "if you don't measure it, you can't fix it". Cummins has shone new light onto the work of, previously mentioned, Dr Joseph Kraft, who developed the "glucose tolerance" test, in the 1960s, a method of testing insulin to show the "insulin status" of an individual or, in other words, their level of insulin resistance. Kraft, a pathologist, measured the insulin status of 14,308 people over 30 years, aged between 8 and 88.

90% Of Those Tested That Resulted as Insulin Resistant Would Be Given a Clear Bill of Health With a Fasting Glucose Test!
The individuals tested with Kraft's method that showed a level of insulin resistance would therefore already be at some point on an undetected journey of inflammatory and/or arterial damage and in need of help or advice. Yet 90% of these same people passed a standard fasting glucose test (the measure for pre-diabetes or diabetes) and would normally be, incorrectly, given a clean bill of health.

A Very Transformative Experiment By A Human Pin Cushion
The other very interesting individual to know about at the moment is Dave Feldman …. a "tour de force" and a one man band of 'self experimentation extraordinaire'. Another engineer that measures at every opportunity. Feldman photographs *everything* he eats and has been testing his cholesterol/lipids to such an extent that he must have become the human pin cushion! He is the founder of cholesterolcode.com and in essence a serial self experimenter. He must have taken more advanced cholesterol tests than anyone else in history. What he has shown in his experiments is staggering because it goes against what we have been told to believe.

A Graph With An Almost Perfect Mirror Image
Over a period of a few days Feldman alternated his meals between high fat and low fat meals. His results consistently showed that he can:

> *lower* his LDL (so called 'bad' cholesterol) by eating *more* fat and
> *raise* his LDL (so called 'bad' cholesterol) by eating *less* fat

LDL cholesterol responds to dietary intake within three days. Feldman could see a very close inversion pattern forming, where a spike in the graph signifying higher fat consumption was mirrored in a drop in the graph for presence of LDL cholesterol. This was consistent over several days. In fact Feldman decided to create an extreme spike in the graph by consuming 349g of fat in a day. This produced the *lowest LDL cholesterol dip* that he had had since being on a low carb, high fat diet.

An Efficient Energy Distribution System
Feldman's work emphasises that cholesterol is a very elegant *energy distribution system* and not a dysfunctional mechanism that needs correcting in increasing numbers of people, with medication.

So If You've Managed It Through This Chapter, What Is The Take-Home Message?
When it comes to cholesterol, lipoproteins and heart disease we have been advised to have a high carbohydrate, low fat diet with plenty of 'heart healthy' grains. We have been sold plenty of 'low fat, healthy' food options that had added sugar for taste

and then told to monitor our cholesterol rather than our insulin. This has been the advice, pretty much since the 1970s. In other words do the wrong thing and look the other way!

Will it turn out that what we should have been doing, all along, was the complete opposite: avoiding vegetable oils that were promoted as healthy and following a higher fat, low carbohydrate diet, avoiding sugar but also grains and monitoring our insulin status instead?

My Shrinking Waist
Judging from the many recent published papers I have researched, the books I have read and the specialists and researchers I have followed …. And the shrinking size of my waist … despite being a middle aged woman …. it is perhaps a little annoying, or should I say tragic, that the official advice has been so very unhelpful.

CHAPTER **10**:   SUGAR UNWRAPPED

Sugar And Disease
If we don't wake up to the harm sugar is causing it has the potential to bankrupt our health service. It is a central cause of the chronic diseases, cancers, pain, suffering and obesity that afflicts most people in this country at some point in their lives.

What About Our Children?
Worse though is what sugar, in the quantities it is consumed in today, is doing to our children. It is our duty to protect them and we are not. In the US, type 2 diabetes in childhood is a growing problem and here in the UK we now see increasing numbers as well and this is generating great alarm.

Where America Goes …. We Follow
Statistical 'bad news' data is impressively worse when it comes to nutrition in America. In the UK today the public health situation may not be as bad but in most things our tendency is to follow America's trend.

Public Enemy Number One
Sugar, and the powerful addiction to it, needs to be treated as public enemy number one with far more vigor and urgency. We cannot wait for government regulations, we must take responsibility for ourselves and our children and we do that by educating ourselves. Addiction to sugar is causing suffering on a grand scale, both physical and mental. It is robbing people of the potential of having a much better quality of life and higher achievement.

Americans in 2012 on average consumed over 18 times more sugar than they did in 1822 from just over 3Kg per year to 60Kg per year (1). *If there are 4g of sugar in a teaspoon then through the food and drinks they consume*
Americans have gone from 4 teaspoons of sugar per day to 41 teaspoons

Wherever We Turn Temptation is There
There are many statistics for the increase of sugar consumption. They are all dramatic but we can see it for ourselves in the western world. Just look at the quantity of fast food, sweet snacks and drinks available and advertised all around us, all the time. We are addicted and we are being "pushed it" constantly.

Sugar should be put out of sight like tobacco. The trouble is it would mean switching the lights off at the supermarket and have us all shopping in the dark!

Sugar Is a Fundamental Cause of Insulin Resistance
Whether or not we appear healthy and thin very many of us are becoming progressively insulin resistant. Yet largely we remain unaware of its significance or the danger. Being knowledgeable about this hormone is vital as it can empower us to avoid:

High blood sugar levels   Dementia   Kidney Failure
Heart Attacks   Mood Swings   Blindness
Strokes   Cancer   Rheumatoid Arthritis
Depression   Alzheimer's   Impotence
Infertility   Sleep Disruption   Lethargy & Fatigue
Multiple Schlerosis   Atheroschlerosis   Autoimmune Disorders
Inflammatory Bowel Disease (2)

We must understand, prevent and reverse Insulin resistance a path to dementia and Alzheimers (also known as Type 3 Diabetes).

Why Do We Still Have Vending Machines in Schools and Hospitals, Where 50% of Clinical Staff Are Obese. … and Why Do Cancer Charities Host Cup Cake Sales as Fundraisers!
We must protect our children. We need to educate ourselves and educate them on the dangers of sugar and stop even more people from making the same mistakes. Insulin resistance starts in childhood but is progressing at a greater rate today due to the excessive amounts of sugar and refined carbohydrates consumed in childhood.

SUGAR, GLUCOSE, FRUCTOSE, FRUIT – WHAT MOST DO NOT KNOW ....

Fructose Affects
The Speed You Age!

SUCROSE known as: Table Sugar, Natural Sugar, Sugar Cane, Sugar Beet
ALL SUCROSE is made up of: 50% Glucose and 50% FRUCTOSE

Why Highlight the Above So Carefully?
Just because something is 'natural' does not mean it is safe.

Fructose Can Put the Speed at Which We Age into Warp Drive (3)
Whereas glucose can be metabolized for energy in all the cells in our body, fructose can only be metabolized by the liver. The scary thing about this fact is the following:

1. Remember that table sugar is 50% glucose/50% fructose.
2. This means that half of the sugar that we eat (ie the glucose) is distributed and processed by 70kg worth of body tissue (an average person's weight) but ....
3. The other half of the sugar (ie the fructose) is only dealt with by about 1.5 kg of tissue in the liver! This shows the extraordinary stress we put on our livers with a diet high in sugar.
4. The excess fructose energy is stored as fat in the liver.
5. A fatty liver is a sick liver. A sick liver means a sick host.

Fructose Drives Insulin Resistance Faster
It is this build up of fat in the liver that drives insulin resistance far faster than glucose does in the rest of the body and explains why we are seeing Type 2 Diabetes occurring much earlier in life, even in our children. Nothing drives a fatty liver faster than high consumption of sweet drinks and fruit juice (even freshly squeezed).

The speed at which fructose creates insulin resistance is why it is becoming more common for us to see many of the inflammatory illnesses that we associate with age manifesting themselves much earlier on in life for those that have a high sugar (fructose) diet, including heart disease and cancer.

Do Not Under Estimate The Speed

In an experiment published in the Journal of Clinical Investigation (April 20, 2009 Havel et al) a group of healthy volunteers were given 25% of their daily caloric intake in the form of a sweetened drink. This was to simulate an average intake of sodas or fruit juice consumed in the population at large. One half of the group's drinks were sweetened with fructose, the other half with glucose. The results were dramatic. In just 6 days the previously healthy 'fructose' group developed insulin resistance and in eight weeks they were diagnosed as pre-diabetic. The 'glucose' group remained relatively unchanged.

If the results were so dramatic in just eight weeks then in just a few years the effects are disastrous. Indeed they are. We are witnessing diabetic mayhem prevailing in all age groups today. Remember that in the past type 2 diabetes used to be referred to as 'age on-set' diabetes. No longer. Our children are in danger and suffering. As adults we should adopt the same attitude towards sugar and our kids as we do with alcohol and smoking.

Don't Be Fooled: Fructose Doesn't Spike Blood Sugar

Ironically fructose used to be considered a good sugar alternative for diabetics because it doesn't show sugar spikes in the blood. No one worried about or tested for insulin resistance build up.

So tackle the fructose in your diet first for dramatic results and then you may want to take a look at the glucose load in your diet in the form of insulin triggering, low nutrient food such as rice, pasta and bread, etc.

Fructose Fast-Tracks The Inflammatory Health Issues
That In The Past Came With Age

Off Guard, We Have Speeded Up Our Ageing Process
Since fructose became so accessible, and not simply available in seasonal fruit, it has become a slow poison and it has caught us off guard. Just because you do not drop dead from it immediately doesn't mean it will not kill you in the end.

Yet Fructose Is A Fundamental Survival Tool In The Animal Kingdom
Fructose provides a fundamental survival mechanism in the animal kingdom and it can be said that it was of great importance to our ancestors' survival in the winter months. ….

Fascinating research in America put a new slant on fructose and concluded that insulin resistance in nature is a normal process not a disease. In fact insulin resistance could be termed a *fat storage condition* essential to the animal kingdom but a precursor to disease for us, in our world today. (4)   The research points out that fructose enables animals, in a matter of weeks, to readily lay down fat stores in their bodies to see them through the winter months.   For example take the hibernating bear …..

Why Bears Have A Sweet Tooth
Bears load up with fructose in the autumn prior to hibernation enabling them to lay down and store substantial, additional fat to normal.   They will consume vast quantities of sweet berries and fruits in the autumn that will contain greater amounts of fructose than earlier in the year when the fruits are less ripe.

This continuous and increased consumption of fructose 'triggers' what is known as metabolic syndrome: insulin resistance, raised fats in the blood, increased abdominal fat, fatty liver and reduced energy levels, all important for their survival through the winter hibernation.

Birds That Fly South in the Winter Load Up with Fructose
Migratory birds increase their fructose consumption to increase their bodies' fat deposits allowing them to survive the long, non-stop flights to sunnier climates.

But Animals Stop Consuming And Humans Just Carry On

The Bears And Birds Burn It Off
In the animal kingdom however the bear effectively fasts over the winter months and the migratory birds burn their fat off during their long, non stop, flights and by the time the spring comes the bear will be lean again.

Humans however, through their ever increasing consumption of fructose have triggered the 'fat switch' activated insulin resistance and metabolic syndrome, but continue to feast on sugar and fruit all year round and make their condition even worse by their over consumption of refined carbohydrates as well.

So fructose continues to be turned into fat in the body, stored and accumulated around the vital organs of a 'thin' person or as belly and/or thigh fat in an obese person.

Spotlight On The Average Modern Western Diet
Should We Be That Surprised So Many Are Estimated to Have Insulin Resistance?

Breakfast's Loaded Sugar and Carb Opportunity
Cereals – Bread – Jam – Pastries - Fruit Juice
Mid Morning Snack's Loaded Sugar and Carb Opportunity
Biscuits – Cake - Chocolate Bars - Coffee or Tea with Sugar - Fizzy Drinks - Crisps
Lunch's Loaded Sugar and Carb Opportunity
Fast Food - Sandwiches - Bread - Crackers - Fruit Juice - Fizzy Drinks - Crisps
Mid Afternoons Loaded Sugar and Carb Opportunity
Crisps - Chocolate Bars - Fizzy Drinks - Dried Fruit
Supper's Loaded Sugar and Carb Opportunity
Pizza - Pasta - Noodles - Rice - Condiments eg ketchup or mayonnaise - Sugar loaded Pre-prepared Meals - Ice Cream - Fizzy Drinks/Alcohol
… And Even the Super Evil Late Evening Snack
Cereal - Chocolate - Biscuits - Hot Sugared Drink

Like a Yo Yo
With feeding patterns like this or similar we are increasing our blood sugars and insulin levels and disrupting our hormones, leading us to feel the need to be in perpetual 'grazing mode', trying to maintain a sugar high so that we don't feel bad. (Headaches, lethargy, anxiety and fuelling the rise of mental health issues).

THE OTHER POWERS OF FRUCTOSE THAT WE MUST TAME

Fructose Disrupts Our Master Hormone Insulin That Leads to the Breakdown in Signalling of the Hormones That Drive Hunger and Fullness

GHRELIN (the "I'm Hungry" Hormone) (5)

Ghrelin is the hormone that is responsible for giving feelings of hunger. Fructose triggers a cascade that stops this hormone from being supressed. So perversely we can continue consuming and remain hungry. The decrease in hunger pangs that Ghrelin can create, will ultimately be our strongest indicator that we have become adapted to easily switching to burning fat and we are on track to regaining our health and re-establishing insulin sensitivity.

PEPTIDE YY (the "I'm Full" Hormone) (6)

It is important to know that the "I'm hungry" hormone Ghrelin, found in the stomach is not responsible for telling us when we are full. That is left to another hormone that is found further down in the intestine and is known as Peptide YY. This hormone kicks in about 20 minutes after we start eating. This time delay is the reason why it is important to eat slowly. If we finish our dish in 10 minutes and want seconds - wait 10 minutes - then decide. Yet even this hormone is disrupted.

Fructose Leads to the Disruption of Leptin Signalling – Leading Our Body to Think It Is Starving When In Fact It Is Overweight (7)

Leptin is a hormone discovered in the 1990s that is formed in the fat cells, so the more fat cells we have the more leptin we have. It is responsible for signalling to the brain that we have enough energy stored in our fat cells. In this situation we will not feel hungry, we will feel energetic and well. The body can afford to be 'liberal' with its energy stores. We feel energized and on top of the world …. Beautiful when all the hormones are in balance ….

Leptin Resistance

However leptin, like insulin, suffers from becoming less efficient and being ignored by the body when levels get too high. So when more and more fat accumulates in the body, leptin presence is increased. This continual production of leptin leads to leptin resistance. In other words, the brain starts to ignore its signals.

The Body Thinks We Are Starving Even Though We Are Constantly Eating
Thus, despite the fact that you are putting on weight and eating plenty of food, the brain, because it is not accepting the Leptin signals, believes it is in starvation mode. The body therefore responds by trying to conserve energy. This gives rise to lethargy and a lack of desire to move. This preference for inactivity is a symptomatic characteristic of obesity. Believing itself to be starving, the body is not so willing to burn its fat stores.

Restoring the hormonal balance that sugar disrupts is key. When achieved it is possible to restore good health, ideal weight and increased vitality. It is a case of:

Get healthy to lose weight
And not
Lose weight to get healthy

Why Eating Fruit is Better Than Drinking Fruit Juice
Fructose in fruit is best consumed with fibre. Eating a high fibre diet is fundamental to health and weight loss as it slows down digestion and gives a feeling of fullness. To illustrate this take the example of a glass of freshly squeezed orange juice. It may easily contain the juice of four oranges. Drinking one glass of orange juice is quick and easy but one would struggle to consume four whole oranges ... and without the fibre in the juice the fructose is rapidly metabolised by the liver and converted to fat. [8]

The 'Speed' of Fructose Intake
A fizzy drink will, on average have 10 teaspoons of sugar with absolutely no fibre in sight to slow down the absorption. The rate at which these are consumed is one of the main driving forces of obesity in the young. Sports Drinks promoted as healthy are often, simply sugared water of some form and can be just as harmful.

Fructose and Non-Alcoholic Fatty Liver Disease
High consumption of sugary drinks and fruit juice, can lead to non-alcoholic fatty liver disease. Unsurprisingly, in communities where alcohol is banned, more soda is consumed and statistics show a higher prevalence of this condition.

Why All "Calories" Are Not Created Equal
It was as recently as the 1980s that new scientific understanding of the effects of fructose emerged, leading to a re-examination of insulin resistance as well.

According to the American pediatric endocrinologist Dr Robert Lustig and author of "Fat Chance", if we eat an extra 150 calories a day of healthy whole foods our risk of diabetes is not affected. If, however, we increase our calories by 150 per day by consuming a sugary drink then our risk of developing diabetes goes up 11 fold. Lustig maintains that calories from other sources can lead to weight gain, calories from sugar uniquely contribute to the risk of type 2 diabetes. Dr Lustig has studied the dangers of fructose and is one of the loudest voices in America, warning of those dangers.

Fructose Feeds the Bad Bugs In Our Digestive Tract
Taking expensive probiotics (good bacteria) whilst still consuming large amounts of sugar may well be a waste of money as sugar will feed our bad bugs and help increase their population and prevent them from being overpowered by our good gut flora/bacteria (responsible in large part for our immune system).

…. And Finally, What About Fructose in Fruit?
After reading all about fructose it wouldn't be surprising if we stayed away! Yet whole fruit is full of very valuable antioxidants, enzymes and fibre that reduce the effect of fructose compared to processed foods and sweet drinks. Eat fruit in moderation especially when trying to lose weight. If you have insulin resistance then eating fruit could stall weight loss. Eat fruit when it is less ripe and antioxidant content is higher and its fructose content is lower. Find out which fruits are higher and lower in fructose. See examples given under "Juicing or Blending". (see page 116).

Fructose and Sunshine (9)
In nature fruit is available when there is an abundance of sunshine, our best source of Vitamin D. Science shows that fructose intake can induce Vitamin D insufficiency. This is not a case for not eating fruit but it shows how clever nature is and as we start to tamper with it (eating bountiful amounts of fruit in the middle of winter) there may be unintended consequences.

Sugar's Canon Balls - A Summary

In Summary Sugar Doesn't Just Fire One Canon Ball At Our Health, It Fires Three

Shot one triggers insulin resistance, diabetes, external obesity and unhealthy, internal fat stores around our organs, leading on to many inflammatory diseases.

Shot two feeds the pathogens (the bad bacteria in our gut) harming the balance of our good gut bacteria that, as we will go on to read, is now believed to make up a staggering 75% of our immune system.

Shot three it depletes your body's store of nutrients especially minerals like magnesium needed to metabolise the sugars and carbohydrates, leaving us deficient in vital nutrients.

Why Sweeteners Are Not a Good Idea (10)

The debate on sweeteners goes backwards and forwards but research is now showing that aspartame may raise insulin and that sweeteners in general cause the body to think it is about to receive sugar and when it doesn't it causes craving. In addition more research is needed on the effect on gut bacteria and indications are that the sweeteners may cause disruption here too.

However there is also another fundamental reason why they are not serving us well. Sweeteners maintain our "sweet tooth". As we reduce our sugar and sweetener consumption our palate will change and we will become more sensitive to the sugar tastes, meaning that, eventually, a little bit of fruit or a tiny teaspoon tip of honey will give us plenty of sugary taste. Not, however, if we keep bombarding our palate with sweeteners.

It's Not the Saturated Fat – It's The Sugar (11)

Sugars in carbohydrates are converted to fats (triglycerides) in the liver; a process known as *lipogenesis.* We should be transplanting from deep in our psyche an image of butter-lined, clogged arteries with an image of bags of sugar transforming themselves from crystals of white purity, labelled 'fat-free' in the packaging to fat of the worst kind, storing itself doggedly around our organs and belly once we consume…. Pure evil.

Is it time to replace the "Low Fat" label with a "No Sugar" One?

CHAPTER 11: AUTOPHAGY

In 2016 the Nobel Prize in Physiology or Medicine went to the Japanese scientist Yoshinori Ohsumi for his discovery of the mechanisms of autophagy. The term *autophagy* comes from auto = self, phagy = eat. It describes a mechanism that eliminates damaged parts of our cells and then recycles healthy components: effectively clearing out pre-cancerous cells, viruses and impaired genes, for example, and reusing healthy parts to build new cells. After infection, autophagy can eliminate invading intracellular bacteria and viruses.

Autophagy acts like a quality control mechanism that is critical for counteracting the negative consequences of ageing but as it slows down, as we get older, it can be assisted. This is because a major way that autophagy is stimulated is through starving the cells and hence why fasting has been shown to have such rejuvenating benefits.

By identifying this process Ohsumi was able to see that the slow down in autophagy as we age can lead to an increase risk of cancer, as well as neurodegenerative disorders such as Parkinsons and Alzheimers.

Autophagy has been known for over 50 years but its fundamental importance in physiology and medicine was only recognized after Yoshinori Ohsumi's paradigm-shifting research in the 1990s.

As research continues in this area we are learning that intermittent fasting, a higher fat, lower carbohydrate diet that enables us to burn fat more often, and short bursts of high intensity exercise, all help activate a regular spring clean of our cells and provide an invaluable cancer prevention strategy.

High levels of insulin in the blood will make it more difficult
for the body to enable autophagy.

CHAPTER 12: PROCESSED FOOD – WHY IT IS BEST AVOIDED

We All Know But Let's Spell It Out

- **Refined Foods:** Such as bread made from refined white flour will have all its nutrients stripped in the processing. Synthetic vitamins reintroduced at a later stage will not function and be bioavailable to the body in the same way as natural wholefoods can offer.

- **Refined Carbohydrates:** Have crept into our diet in such quantities, they are generally low fibre foods and lead to constant blood sugar surges and that lead down a road to insulin resistance, diabetes and feed the bad bacteria in our gut.

- **Sugar and High Fructose Corn Syrup:** It is inescapable. Western society adds sugar to tea, coffee, canned drinks, fruit juice, squashes, puts it in cereal … puts it on top of cereal … adds it to yoghurts and savoury food and savoury sauces not to mention the oceans of biscuits, cakes, breads, sweets, chocolate etc, etc … Adding sugar to processed food increases its shelf life.

- **Processed Foods are Made to Press All Your Buttons:** Leaving you wanting more and more and more. The food manufacturer's aim is to produce "hyper-rewarding" products that leave you totally addicted.

- **Heating:** Most processed foods undergo heat treatment that generally destroys heat sensitive vitamins and damages unstable cooking oils.

- **Vegetable Oil:** is used in most processed foods as it is much cheaper than animal fat but it is high in Omega 6 and our over consumption of it leads to chronic inflammation when not balanced with Omega 3. The heated polyunsaturated fat of vegetable oils can lead to inflammation and disease.

- **Preservatives, Flavourings, Colour, Texture Enhancing Chemicals:**
- The more chemicals are added to a food the harder your body will have to work in order for it to metabolise and get rid of those chemicals. These foods do not add value but use up nutrients in your body that could be used to enhance and protect you instead.

- **Low in Fibre:** A common characteristic of most chemically processed food is that it is low in fibre.

- **Deodorising:** Due to the processing of food some items will actually go rancid and the resulting unpleasant smells need to be disguised through deodorising techniques. An example of this can occur in the processing of vegetable oils. [1]

- **Quality:** Due to the very nature of processing the initial whole foods selected to be included in the final processed article is unrecognisable and the quality can be compromised. For example foods containing processed meats.

- **Storage and Transit:** From the moment fresh food is picked it starts to lose many of its beneficial nutrients. The longer the food spends in transit and storage the less benefit it is likely to offer you.

CHAPTER 13:   IGNORING THE MICROBIOME

Our Fear Of Bugs Could Be Killing Us (1)
Do you know who you really are?
Healthy humans have around 100, 000,000,000,000 (that's 100 trillion microbes) in their gut.

The gut alone contains 10 times more of these microbes than human cells in the rest of our body put together.

So it can be said that 90% of what we are is effectively a constantly evolving and changing mass of bugs! Known as our microbiome, microbiota, microflora, gut flora, gut bacteria or simply bugs in our gut.

That thought on its own is as empowering as it is frightening…..

Empowering because if you get sick then you really do have a chance through good food and good choices to get well again. Wholesome, nutrient dense food has enormous beneficial power on the bugs in your gut. Frightening because all the bad habits and toxic lifestyles we pursue also have very fundamental and negative impacts on us. Our bugs are constantly evolving and responding to our food and lifestyle choices including stress and sleep.

The Difference Between Genes and Bacteria – Quite A Lot I Hope ….
We, and our chimpanzee friends share an almost identical set of genes (99%)! What makes us different is our bacteria. We have a huge variety of bacteria, chimps don't. (1426 varieties of pathogens and parasites in humans versus 37 in chimps, with 28 shared varieties).

Are You Too Clean? – You Might Not Want to Wash Those Bugs Away!
Our obsession with cleanliness and the use of antibacterial wipes and sprays means that our immediate environment is more sterile than, it now appears, it ought to be. These habits and others that we pursue to eradicate bacteria around us could be causing us much more serious problems than we realise. We are predominantly a mass of bugs and it is apparently very important for us to be much more

interconnected with the bugs in the outside world that bring us healthy microbial diversity. If we feed ourselves properly we strengthen the many good microbial communities in our gut that protect us from the rogue pathogens.

How Should Your Microbes Work For You

I say 'should' because many of us are actively doing things that weaken our microbiota or 'gut flora' and in turn weakening ourselves (that I will highlight later).

Our gut flora should work to give us:
- Our protective immune system (around 75% of it is controlled by our gut flora).
- Protection from infection
- Healthy regulation of our metabolism
- Good digestive health
- Vitamins and compounds created by our gut flora for healthy body function
- Mental clarity and good brain function.
- Help reduce our potential for inflammation by protecting us from the damage we inflict through our poor lifestyle choices

A neglected microbiota can eventually wreak havoc on our bodies.

Microbes Rule

The greater the variety of good bugs you have in your gut the healthier you are likely to be

Although there have been pockets of understanding throughout the ages of this topic, it has largely gone ignored and misunderstood in recent history. It can even be said that such things as pasteurisation, refrigeration, disinfectants and antibiotics have not served us as well as we may have thought. These features have put a barrier between us and the microbial world. It is becoming apparent, instead, that the more access we have to the vast array of bugs around us the more diversity of bugs we build up in our gut. That, it now transpires, is the secret of good health.

Our Well Intentioned Actions Have Been Disrupting This Amazing System That Has Taken All of History to Evolve

The use of antibiotics is just one example of how we have been inadvertently altering this delicate microbiotic system. For antibiotics act indiscriminately going in to kill the good bugs that we rely on for good health as well as the bad bugs.

So although antibiotics have protected, for example, millions of children from dying from infectious diseases over the past 70 years, in the long term the use of antibiotics may be contributing to a fundamental change to the effectiveness and strength of our microbiota. This diminishing strength has translated as a diminished strength in our collective immune systems that has lead to the advent of an ever more common feature of modern illness – Autoimmune Disease. (2)

Listing Auto Immune Disorders Gives a Snap Shot of our Modern World:

- Type 1 Diabetes
- Allergies
- Lupus
- Autism
- Sjogren's Syndrome
- Fibromyalgia
- Colitis
- Crohns Disease
- Chronic Fatigue Syndrome
- Rheumatoid Arthritis
- Coeliac Disease
- Aspergers
- Multiple Sclerosis
- Graves Disease
- Psoriasis
- Hashimoto's Thyroiditis
- Inflammatory Bowel Disease

Autism and The Gut/Brain Axis

There is rapidly developing interest in the gut/brain axis as the conditions along the autism spectrum appear to be increasing. (3) Here too, it seems that, whilst a lot of attention is given to coping with the symptoms of autism with management techniques, not enough, if any, attention is given to the possible gut dysbiosis (microbial imbalance) that may exist and be causing or worsening the condition in individuals with autism. In this area the neurologist and nutritionist Dr Natasha Campbell McBride wrote a comprehensive account of her learning experience in helping her own autistic son, the nutritional protocol she developed and the clinical experiences she gained with patients she went on to treat. Her work was published in 2010 in the book "Gut and Psychology Syndrome – Natural Treatment for Autism, Dyspraxia, ADD, ADHD, Dyslexia, Depression and Schizophrenia".

What Is Weakening Our Immunity?
Things That Are Said to Be Weakening Our Gut Flora/Immune System

Antibiotics	Disinfectant sprays	Caesarian births
Steroids	The Pill	Pollution
Chemicals	Toxins	Pharmaceuticals
Anti acids	Antibacterial gels	Processed foods

Sugar - as this will feed the pathogens/bad bugs that go toward tipping the balance of good bugs to bad in your gut.

Even immensely beneficial aspects like clean water, sanitation and the pasturisation of milk, although life-saving, have also impacted in the long term to leave us less robust and open to new autoimmune conditions that were less prevalent before. I think the expression is we have borrowed from Peter to pay Paul …..

Weakening of Our Immune Systems Down Our More Recent Generations
After a number of generations these recent social changes and habits have slowly altered and reduced the number of beneficial microbes that our grandmothers were able to pass on, through breast feeding and natural childbirth, to our mothers who in turn passed on to us and we then passed onto our children. With each generation the gut bacteria became slightly weaker than before.

So it is that today many more children seem to be born with allergies and develop asthma, autism and many other conditions that may not simply be being diagnosed due to 'better diagnosis techniques' but possibly because of ever weakening immune systems due to diminished gut flora being passed down the generations.
In 2005 an estimated 5,658,900 had been diagnosed with Asthma (approximately 1 in 9 of the population). Approximately 32,577,300 prescriptions were issued for the condition in 2005 alone. (4) In 1927 when the Asthma Research Council, now known as Asthma UK was founded there were estimated to be around 200,000 cases of asthma in the UK.

Spotlight on Caesarian Sections

One of the most fundamental ways that our microbes (and inherent immune system) pass down the generations is through the birthing process. The microbes that a baby ingests, and its skin is covered in, during its exit through the birth canal are invaluable. Notably the lactobacilli flourishes in the mother's vagina during pregnancy and makes the birth canal more acidic giving powerful protection against the more alkali-loving pathogens.

A mother's water's breaking is a far more significant event than most of us appreciate. As the waters splash onto the mother's thighs it spreads the bacteria, that the waters have swept up, as it came through the vagina. The Lactobacilli is transported onto the mother's skin and colonises her entire skin surface extremely quickly. By the time the baby makes contact with it's mother's skin and suckles on her nipples nature has not only ensured a safe, pathogen free environment for the new born but also that the baby incorporates this age-old and vital microbe into its own immune system.

Not To Be Elected Lightly

Caesarian sections can be life saving for both the mother and child in some cases but today we see it, perhaps, being offered too easily, without mothers understanding the true costs. By not passing through the birth canal, a baby born by C-section may not be starting life with the same advantages of a baby born naturally. In addition, due to surgery, it is probable that the mother receives antibiotics in the process adding to the impact of microbial loss.

All is not lost for those children who are born by C section as good diet and the right foods can go a long way to address the disadvantage. Yet disadvantage it may well, scientifically, turn out to be and these children may be more prone to allergies, asthma, ear infections as they grow. (5) In more enlightened hospitals, techniques are becoming available to minimise this microbial loss to babies born by C-section.

How Can We Strengthen Our Gut Flora And Then Our Immune System

List of things that could benefit our gut flora:

- **Owning a dog!**
- **Gardening**
- **Opening the windows** … and letting fresh air and a fresh exchange of bugs into our highly insulated, double glazed homes and offices.
- **Probiotics** can help to increase the number of good bacteria in your gut. Sources: fermented food eg yogurt, sauerkraut, cheese. Homemade fermented food can provide much more potent forms of probiotics than the probiotic capsules available over the counter.
- **Prebiotics ie Fibre** on the other hand, are food sources that do not add bacteria directly but rather serve to feed existing bacteria in the gut and strengthen your immune system. Sources: Fibre, including fermentable resistant starch found in beans, vegetables and other plant based foods. Our bugs benefit from feeding off the fibre and the polyphenol phytonutrients that are bound to the fibre. (6)
- **Phytonutrients -** there are more than 4,000 of these compounds that we know of to date found in plant foods. Very many of them are antioxidants that counteract the damaging effects of free radicals in our body. They can protect against inflammation and reduce tumour growth. They are responsible for the strong flavours and bright colours in plant foods and help plants defend themselves from insect attack.

Examples:

Allicin in garlic, onions, leeks	Resveratrol in red wine
Quercetin in citrus fruits, apples, onions	Curcumin in turmeric
Capsaicin in chilli and paprika	Rosmarinic acid in rosemary
Sage	Thyme
Peppermint	Oregano

Faecal transplants ……. Don't recoil in horror, this process is generating more and more interest. It has been used to successfully treat people in hospital. More people today, after an operation, have even further weakened immunity and are more likely to develop an infection known as C Difficile. This infection has had a lot of coverage in the media. It is a notoriously difficult and dangerous pathogen to treat that has been developing resistance to antibiotics. But patients who have been treated through the use of faecal transplants for this infection have nearly all been cured (96%). The transplant will come from a donor who has a healthy profile of bugs living in their intestine that can fight off C Difficile. (7)

Unintended Consequences
There have, however, been reported case studies of individuals who have received faecal transplants and have dramatically changed body shape. By receiving gut bacteria from someone that has a tendency to be overweight can alter the physical shape of the recipient. This has been observed frequently in mice. It is an observation that may have consequences in the future to treat depression.

Obesity and Antibiotics
There is a growing school of thought that there is a link between obesity and our individual make up of microbes in our gut. Two main aspects to shed light on are:

Antibiotics
Farmers have known for over 50 years that giving farm animals such as cattle low dose antibiotics increases their weight and therefore their value in meat weight. The antibiotics change the structure of the microbiota in the host that can lead to a metabolic, immune and hormonal imbalance that leads to weight gain. Our consumption of these foods together with our own personal cases of antibiotic intake, especially in childhood may be another factor that has contributed towards the obesity epidemic in modern society.

Firmicutes and Bacteriodetes
Although we can have thousands of different types of bacteria in and on our bodies there are two main 'family' groups that these diverse bacteria come under – Firmicutes and Bacteriodetes. If you have not heard these two words yet you will … a lot! There are about 50 phyla or 'family groups' of bacteria that we know of in the world today. Of the fifty 'phyla', six of these make up 99.9% of all the bacteria in and on your body and these include the two largest groups, Firmicutes and the Bacteriodetes.

A landmark study by Harvard University wanted to analyse the difference in microbial characteristics of 15 healthy children in the European Union and 14 healthy children in a rural African village called Burkina Faso. The study has become so famous that it is often just referred to as the Burkina Faso study. What the study showed was that the African children had a much higher ratio of Bacteriodetes compared to Firmicutes and the European children were the other way round with a much higher ratio of Firmicutes.

Importantly the Bacteriodetes in the African community were able to maximise their energy intake from fibre and were protected from inflammation and intestinal diseases. Their diet was low in fat and animal protein and rich in fibre, starch and vegetables They were on average breast-fed until the age of two compared to one year in the European children. From then onwards the European children's diet was rich in fat, protein and sugar and low in fibre particularly resistant starches. This diet is associated with a rapid increase in intestinal diseases. [8]

Altering Your Ratio
In the Harvard study they stated that 'it was reasonable to surmise that an increase in the Firmicutes to Bacteriodetes ratio in European children, probably driven by …. diet, might predispose them to future obesity. This F/B ratio may also be considered a useful obesity biomarker. '

High levels of Firmicutes appear, therefore, not be desirable, since they may alter the behaviour of our genes and trigger inflammation, diabetes, poor heart health as well as obesity. [9]

The Microbiome is Even More ….
We have been lead to believe that our genes come from the sperm and egg of our parents. It would appear that in reality about 23,000 genes[10] come from our parents but the bacteria in our gut is thought to account for around 3 million more genes! This is one of the reasons why the study of Epigenetics is showing us that we have far more control than we previously thought over our health. Our lifestyle and dietary choices have significant influence over whether or not we trigger our genes and become ill or remain healthy.

A very good article introducing the Microbiome to readers in The Economist magazine of August 18, 2012 wrote:

".... Evolution has aligned the interests of host and bugs.
In exchange for raw materials and shelter the microbes that
live in and on people feed and protect their hosts, and are thus
integral to that host's well-being. Neither wishes the other harm."

Time to Rethink Our "War" on Bugs
Science is swinging round today, in a quite dramatic way, back to the importance of the Microbiome, gut health and our whole approach to our 'war' on bugs.

Caution and Balance and a New Type of Medicine
When it comes to the microbiome the phrase 'one size fits all' certainly does not apply. The microbiome shows us just how different we are to each other and a reason why we all react differently to our environment, foods and medication.

As our knowledge of the microbiome evolves there is also more understanding that the so called 'bad bugs' (pathogens) are not necessarily out and out 'bad'. Take the pathogen H Pylori – it is well known to the medical community. The general approach to date is that if you have it in your gut it is best treated to remove it. However recent studies have shown that in fact H Pylori may be a good thing to have in youth as it may help protect children against asthma. In fact research conducted through statistical analysis showed that individuals with H Pylori were 40% less likely to develop asthma.

Therefore another contributing factor for the increased incidence of asthma today may be due to the fact that with better sanitation and hygiene in general, it is less likely that this age old pathogen, which has been passed down the generations, is not as prevalent amongst humans as it once was.

In older people however H Pylori can go on to produce problems such as reflux, ulcers and stomach cancer.

Perhaps the case of H Pylori offers, in fact, a good example of how medicine may evolve in the future as we become more knowledgeable in the field of gut bacteria. Doctors may be able to add or remove strains of bacteria in order to prevent or cure individual conditions. (11)

Repair Your Gut And Strengthen Immunity
Probiotics foods: Supply your intestine with trillions of beneficial bacteria, especially from fermented foods.

Prebiotic foods: Supply the beneficial bacteria already living in your intestine with the plant foods it needs to thrive

Probiotic Food and The Forgotten Art of Fermentation
Before refrigeration was invented fermentation was the method used for thousands of years, by people all over the world, to preserve and store food for months/years. Examples of these foods range from alcohol, cheese, sauerkraut, yoghurt, kefir, kimchi and many, many more, as just about anything can be fermented.

Fermented food is an extremely valuable but lost art in western society. It provides the body with huge amounts of beneficial good bacteria for a healthy digestive system leading to a strong immune system. To give you an idea of the strength and value of say, a good, homemade sauerkraut, a teaspoon can provide you with millions more beneficial bacteria than several packets of probiotic tablets.

War
There is an on-going war between the good bacteria in your gut that keeps you healthy, strong and mentally agile and the bad bugs (pathogens) that live there too. Pathogens thrive on sugar and other refined carbohydrates whilst probiotic fermented foods have the ability to radically increase the population of good bugs thus driving out the pathogens from your gut. (12)

In recent years with the emphasis on bacteria being viewed as simply dangerous, something to be eliminated by antibiotics or antibacterial sprays, the importance of this bacterial balance in the gut has been severely underestimated and even avoided. Fear of bacteria meant that we became unsure of the safety of fermented foods.

We Become Sick When the Pathogens Win the War
In today's sugar-laden society pathogens have the upper hand as we are busy feeding them exactly what they need to thrive. We must take on board once more, as people knew in the past, that in order to have good physical and mental health we must first fix our digestive health.

Sauerkraut and cheeses made from raw milk are my favourite options but there are many options and much written on the subject for you to explore and choose from. I used "The Complete Idiot's Guide to Fermenting Foods" by Wardeh Harmon that set me quickly on a successful and tasty path. In fact my favourite is sauerkraut adding leeks, fennel, fennel seeds and dill to my cabbage as I love the licorice flavour but the guide encourages you to experiment. It also explains why the fermentation process is safe.

Exploding Jars at the Supermarket
With the advent of supermarkets, properly fermented vegetables were no longer so viable to sell. Fermentation is an on-going process that produces perfectly safe gaseous by-products but trying to place fermenting sauerkraut on a supermarket shelf would probably result in exploding jars! Fermented vegetables have the same sour, vinegary flavour as modern day pickled vegetables that you do find on the supermarket shelf. These items however are not the product of fermentation but recipes using vinegar itself to provide that same tangy taste to complement meat dishes. Most health benefits are lost though.

Like chicken stocks and bone broth, this is a food item that is easy to prepare at home and can be made, literally, by the bucket load and stored in special pickling jars, that will last for months and months. Remember even just a teaspoon a day is enough to give the immune system a massive boost. I like to eat mine as a condiment with cheese.

Captain Cook and Scurvy

Finally and to press the point home of how marvelous sauerkraut is, it also provides potent anti-inflammatory benefits and is high in Vitamin A and C. In fact sauerkraut can contain up to 200 times more Vitamin C than the original vegetables used to make it.

It was this fact that lead Captain Cook the famous explorer of the 18th century to introduce it as a long term storable foodstuff on board his ships to provide his sailors with Vitamin C during their epic journeys across the world. He thereby prevented the long-standing problem of scurvy suffered, often fatally, by those embarking on these journeys where fresh food was unobtainable. For this, Captain Cook was awarded the Copley Gold Medal in 1776 by the Royal Society.

CHAPTER 14: SPOTLIGHT ON PHYTONUTRIENTS

The Benefits of Plant Foods
Scientists are continuing to identify unique, plant-based phytonutrients. The phytonutrient message is aim for colour variety.

Plant based foods contain over 4,000 groups of different phytonutrients. These compounds are responsible for, amongst other things, the bright colours and strong aromatic flavours. Phytonutrients are important in preventing and fighting cancer. (1)

Variety and Availability
Greater variety of plant foods enhances health. Phytonutrients in plants provide us with many types of valuable anti-oxidants. Their richest sources are sometimes in the skin of the plant so peeling can remove much of the health benefit. Phytonutrient content may be highest at the food's freshest time; cooking can reduce the benefits of these compounds.

Target Colour
Phytonutrients are divided into five colours: Green, Red, White, Purple/Blue and Yellow/Orange.

Red Foods
For Heart, DNA, Prostate And Urinary Tract Health
Well known example:
Lycopene Source: Cooked Tomatoes

Orange/Yellow Foods
For Eye And Immune Health, Supporting Growth And Development
Well known examples:
Alpha-carotene Source: pumpkin, carrots for cardiovascular health
Beta-carotene Source: peppers – cos or romaine lettuce, kale.

Purple/Blue Foods
For Brain And Cognitive Health And Heart, Arteries, Bone. Protects Against Cancers And Ageing Effects.
Well known example:
Resveratrol Source: Red wine

Green Foods
For Eye & Gum Health, Lung, Liver, Arterial & Cell Function. Protects Against Cancers
Well known example:
Lutein/Zeaxanthin Source: Kale – Spinach- Paprika

White Foods
For Bone, Circulatory And Heart Health And Arterial Function. Protects Against Cancer.
Well Known example:
Allicin Source: Garlic – onions – leeks
Quercetin Source: onions – citrus fruits – apples

Top Tip To Make You Tip Top
Garlic but specifically Allicin in garlic can act as an effective, natural antibiotic but it also has certain anti-viral and anti-fungal and anti-cancer properties.

Allicin has been shown to prevent blood clotting by 90%, in a study it was a "significantly more potent platelet inhibitor than aspirin at nearly equivalent concentrations." (2) Although it is not rich in vitamins and minerals it has a wealth of healing traits that has made it valuable and sought after throughout history.

Top Tip
Allicin is the crucial health-giving enzyme and it is only formed when the garlic is crushed and alliin and alliinase enzymes merge to produce allicin. In addition to this, one must wait a few minutes before heating the garlic otherwise the heat sensitive allinase is destroyed before it can create the allicin and you risk missing all its benefits. So when we start cooking we should always crush our garlic first and set it aside for 10 minutes to work its magic.

Get Excited About Herbs And Spices (3)

We can tell by their flavour that they pack an extra big punch. We should use every opportunity to incorporate and combine them into our cooking, whether it is soups, salads, vegetable or meat or fish dishes.

The goodness of herbs and spices is highly concentrated and alternating and maintaining variety is important. Incorporating these regularly into our cooking is a great thing to do.

Let's remind ourselves of some of them, some of the most powerful are:

Spices	Curcumin/Turmeric	Ginger	Coriander seeds
	Fennel Seeds	Chilli	Carraway
	Saffron	Cardamon	Black Pepper
	Cayenne Pepper	Paprika	Cloves
	Nutmeg	Cumin	Star Anise
	Capers	Cinnamon	Curry Powder

Herbs	Basil	Parsley	Dill
	Marjoram	Rosemary,	Coriander
	Thyme	Tarragon	Oregano
	Fennel	Sage	Peppermint

Not to mention all the wonderful aromatic flavours in Thai and south east Asian cooking …..

Like everything else – it is good to alternate the herbs and spices we use and be generous when cooking with them!

…. And What About Nuts?

Nuts are rich in vitamins, minerals, fibre, antioxidants and other bioactive polyphenols. They also contain monounsaturated fats and polyunsaturated fats (enough Omega 6 can be consumed from moderate nut consumption and Omega 6 should be kept to a minimum in additional sources).   Be wary of nut flours such as almond flour as it may be too concentrated and too easy to over consume almonds (a cup of almond flour can contain approximately 90 almonds).

For a Concentrated Intake of Phytonutrients: Juicing Or Blending?
Juicing and blending have the potential to be very useful ways of enhancing our intake of nutrients in a day and of making it easier to consume our 5,7 or 10 a day! However, we must be wary of the fructose and keep our blood sugar levels stable.

Blending
For an extra hit of fibre and nutrients in a raw form the blended smoothie is becoming increasingly popular. It is becoming the prevalent opinion that when consuming fruit it is better to go with the blending option not juicing, as blending will retain the fibre of the fruit and slow down the absorption of the fructose sugar.

Fresh tasting, raw vegetable smoothies are being enjoyed by more and more people. The use of cucumber, celery, mint cleverly disguise too much of a 'green' flavour and when combined with flavoursome berries, spices and other herbs, the latest smoothie recipes are really worth trying.

Juicing
The advantage that juicing is said to have over blending is that with the fibre removed, the nutrients in the juice have the capacity to be more fully and quickly absorbed through the gut wall. With vegetable juicing this speed and ease of absorption is enhanced and has the potential to act as a fantastic natural supplement/boost of vitamins, minerals and antioxidants.

However, when it comes to fruit, juicing needs to be moderated. Adding apples, pears and other high fructose fruits to your juices will only go to raise your blood sugars too quickly as all the fibre that can go towards tempering that blood sugar high has been removed.

Finally, and a bit of a blow to juicing, we are discovering that the majority of phytonutrients may be bound to fibre providing further incentive to either eat the whole fruit or vegetable or blend it, to maintain all possible health benefits. (4)

"Swill It Around A While"
Whatever one chooses, juicing or blending, the important thing to remember is that the first stage of digestion occurs in the mouth. When drinking a smoothie or a juice it is important to keep it in the mouth and "swill it around a while" as the enzyme called Amylase that is secreted in the mouth is responsible for the initial digestion of carbohydrate. Allowing smoothies or juices through to our digestive system without being properly digested can cause an array of health issues.

Let's Be Wary of the Fructose Content of the Fruits We Choose to Use
As they contain between 5-10g of fructose per medium portion size, look out for the fructose content of:

mangoes	grapes	cherries
apples	pears	bananas

Fruits listed below only contain between 0.2g-3.5g of fructose per medium portion. (USDA National Nutrient Database).

lime	lemon	cranberries
plums	grapefruit	peaches
raspberries	kiwis	oranges

116

CHAPTER 15:   HOW MUCH FIBRE DO WE REALLY NEED?

The Characteristics of Fibre
- Fibre comes from plant foods.
- Fibre is either insoluble or soluble, non-fermentable or fermentable.
- Resistant starch is also classified as a fibre. Named for its ability to resist digestion in the small intestine and slowly ferment in the large intestine, thus feeding the healthy gut bacteria that do not produce gas so do not cause bloating.
- A high fibre diet will slow down the absorption of sugars, avoiding spikes in blood sugars and reducing insulin stimulation.

Resistant Starch - Fermentable Fibre
Sources: Legumes, nuts and seeds, starchy vegetables and fruits such as green bananas, sweet potatoes, oats, cooked and cooled potatoes and rice.

Resistant starch is "resistant" to digestion as the name implies. Normally enzymes in the small intestine breakdown starches into sugar, instead resistant starch travels down the gut and is still intact in the colon where good bacteria feeds on it. This beneficial fermentation process produces *Butyrate,* a short chain fatty acid (SCFA) that strengthens your brain and gut. Butyrate is found in high amounts in healthy, butter from pasture fed cows (hence the word 'butyrate').

Sometimes We Need a Bacterial Spring Clean
Those that have been fortunate enough to have been born by natural birth, been breast fed for a reasonable amount of time, managed to avoid antibiotics (especially in infancy), and have avoided medications, especially anti acids and have eaten healthily, will have a good chance of being hosts of a good microbiome. However, those that have highly inflamed intestines through the consumption of a poor diet and not benefitting from the above, may need to avoid fibre for a while. This is because the consumption of sugar and refined grains can lead to a build up of bad bugs (pathogens). These types of bugs create gas, bloating, irritation and weaken your immunity amongst other things. Embarking on a ketogenic diet and restricting large amounts of fibre and carbohydrates for a period allows the starvation of these bad bugs.

Good Guys Produce Butyrate The Bad Guys are Just Full of Hot Air …
Once this has occurred, a combination of probiotics, to 'reseed' your gut with healthy bacteria should be followed up with a diet with ample vegetables and goods levels of fibre to nurture and grow the seeds. Avoiding sugar and low fibre carbohydrates is important as you do not want to allow a re-colonisation of bad bacteria again. An absence of gas in your digestive system is a good indicator that your gut is healthier and the good guys are winning.

Rebuilding New and Healthy Cultures
Once this bacterial clear out has occurred it is important to rebuild new and varied cultures of good bacteria. This is best done with the consumption of fermented vegetables that provide probiotics and prebiotics simultaneously, together with a variety of high fibre, low carbohydrate vegetables.

High Fibre, Low Carbohydrate Vegetables

Artichokes	Onions	Garlic	Broccoli	Brussel Sprouts
Leeks	Avocado	Courgettes	Cabbage	Lettuce
Spinach	Swiss Chard	Asparagus	Fennel	Celery
Cauliflower	Mushrooms			

Do not be tempted to stick to one source, it is important to alternate and keep your diet diverse and seasonal.

Fibre Can Limit Nutrient Absorption
It may be the case that fibre may have some harmful side-effects that are easy to overcome when healthy but become a burden when sick. For example it has been proposed that absorption of nutrients through the gut wall takes time but fibre speeds up the passage of food through the intestine, perhaps preventing better absorption of nutrients. Meat, for instance takes time to process as most of it is digested and used by the body, if eaten with fibre it can be 'pushed' through at a faster rate meaning that the body may not benefit from all the nutrients it has to offer. In addition some fibre even binds with minerals preventing absorption altogether.

Bowel Issues

For those with Irritable Bowel Syndrome and other gut disorders such as Crohns and colitis, it may prove beneficial to replace fibrous vegetables, wholegrains and rough brans with broths, healthy fats and fermented vegetables, or even just a period of time eating only meat (this acts as a full-on elimination diet whilst still allowing nutrification)! Those that pursue these approaches are seeing better results with a calming of the gut wall and better nutritional uptake. The amino acids in bone broth plus the good gut bacteria generated by fermented vegetables and the increase of more bioavailable vitamins in animal fats and meat enable those with damaged gut wall linings to heal whilst enabling better absorption of vitamins, minerals and nutrients.

Fibre is a Good Example of A Topic That May See A Lot of Reassessment

The more we learn about our gut bacteria the more we realise that the topic of fibre is complex. It is not good enough, as we have seen, to just aim for lots of roughage. Lectins in certain plant foods may be problematic, causing further possible irritation to an already inflamed gut. Seasonal variation in vegetables may also prove to be beneficial allowing for a greater variety of healthy bacteria.

Do We Need to Eat Grains to Reach Our Recommended Intake of Fibre?

The approximate recommendation of fibre intake is 30g per day. To reach this target we are advised to include grains and starchy vegetables, yet this leads to a level of carbohydrate and sugar consumption that does not allow us to sustain a low insulin status lifestyle.

Those that claim that a low carbohydrate diet does not provide enough fibre need, perhaps, to look again. Since vegetables, nuts and seeds are able to provide ample fibre whilst still keeping our calories, carbs and sugar intake low enough to maintain healthy insulin levels. In addition these sources are richer in vitamins, minerals and other micronutrients. It may be for this reason that people who eat vegetables but also meat, eggs and dairy, are healthy, irrespective of fibre consumption.

Do We Need Lots and Lots of Fibre?

There is no evidence that supports the recommended 30g of fibre per day will make us healthier. Perhaps it is just the case that those that aim to achieve higher fibre intake are also mindful of other healthy lifestyle options that result in better health for those individuals. However, those that challenge the notion of the need for high fibre intake, will have a hard time. Yet with unhealthy modern diets it can certainly be argued that once you have seeded your gut with pathogens, then too much fibre may lead to further inflammatory irritation. Once we have re-seeded our gut with foods such as kefir, fermented vegetables and raw cheeses, how much fibre do we need to consume to be healthy? Only we can assess that by monitoring our own bowel movement changes and general health. Perhaps we would do better if we focused on the nutrient density of our food instead of our fibre intake? For nutrient density, meat, eggs and dairy will win every time.

The Recommended Levels of Fibre Intake Wax and Wane Over the Decades

Books and individuals appear that shift the thinking. Today we are still greatly influenced by the observations of Dr Dennis Burkitt and his vivid advocacy of the fibre hypothesis. In 1979, fibre became a top topic with the publication of Burkitt's book *"Don't Forget Fibre in Your Diet"*. In it, Burkitt noted that rural black Africans suffered very little cancer of the colon. He concluded that their high fibre diet meant that food travelled faster through the intestine promoting better cleansing of the gut and less likelihood of cancer generating conditions.

Yet we must remember that rural Africans have had many other advantages over industrialised communities; less pollution, toxins, stress, junk food, etc. It is also worth noting that there were other communities also that experienced low colon cancer levels, and disease in general, whilst eating a low-fibre diet, such as the Massai tribe in Africa and the Inuit of the far Northern Hemisphere.

If We Do Not Eat Junk, Perhaps, We Do Not Need Fibre to Slow Down the Absorption of Sugars

It is, of course, true that fibre will slow down the absorption of glucose and other sugars. Yet if we reject refined foods and eat foods that spare insulin, such as meat, eggs and dairy, we will avoid this issue altogether.

Is There a Need for Speed?

High fibre diets enable faster transit of food through the gut. This has been viewed as beneficial. Yet, as mentioned, animal foods take longer to break down and digest, as all parts are absorbed and used by the body. Thus it may be the case that too much fibre does not allow the body enough time to digest, absorb and benefit from all the nutrients animal foods provide, before being swept through by dietary fibre, and excreted. An idea of rotting food "lingering" in the gut has instilled fear of cancer. Yet should this image be questioned, what is the evidence? If the food being eaten is cancerous, perhaps the best thing to do is to stop eating that food!

Cleansing Our Bowels

Vegetables will produce ample fibre to "sweep up" our bowels but the fasting process also provides time for the bowels to empty and rest.

In the End Where Is Fibre Nirvana?

What are the signals we can use to assess whether we have reached a good balance of fibre intake:

Good overall health
Regular, healthy bowel movements
Less gas and bloating
Less inflammation
Less need for …. toilet paper …. (Sorry!!)

CHAPTER 16: LECTINS – PLANT DEFENCE SYSTEMS AND US

What Are Lectins?
Lectins are poisonous plant proteins (of different strengths) designed to protect plants from being eaten at certain times. In nature animals and insects are quite tuned in to 'when' to eat certain plants and 'which' plants to avoid – but are we?

Recently lectins have a made a big 'come back' into general discourse thanks to an interesting book published in 2017 called "The Plant Paradox" by Dr Steven Gundry.

Gluten
One of the most famous and commonly problematic lectins. I choose to avoid gluten, though not completely, in case I build up an unnecessarily serious intolerance. (2)

Lectins Can Become Unwelcome Invaders
Plants have lectins of different strengths that may also increase and subside in their life cycle. Lectins are not digestible by humans and they can enter the blood stream unchanged. Most lectins will not kill us though, legumes, for example can cause severe food poisoning or even kill if they are not pre-soaked and prepared properly before consuming. Over a lifetime, however, an on-going, low-grade assault on our bodies by plant lectins can prove to be unwelcome invaders. They create inflammatory, immune system responses in our bodies that eventually make us ill with symptoms such as skin rashes and joint pain.

Lectins can cause flatulence and diarrhoea. Those suffering from systemic inflammation can have symptoms worsen with some lectin containing foods.

Searching for the Rogues
The concept of an "elimination" diet looks at removing some of these lectin-rich foods, to see whether they are having an adverse effect on individuals. Some common examples are:

Grains, beans, legumes, lentils, peanuts and cashews as they carry the most lectins. In addition, other examples to point out are the nightshade family, aubergines, tomatoes, potatoes, peppers, etc.

However preparing beans and legumes in a pressure cooker will eliminate most of the problem. In addition tomatoes, squash, pumpkins and courgettes should be peeled and deseeded.

My Neapolitan Grandmother Knew All This ….
A once common piece of kitchen equipment in Italy was a saucepan/sieve that had a handle coming up from the inside base with which you would rotate two blades. This was used extensively to prepare tomatoes for the copious amount of tomato sauce used in Italian cooking. The blades would breakdown the tomatoes allowing the juice to flow through the sieve, separating out the seeds and skin that were known to cause digestive issues if eaten in quantity. This thick juice is known as *passata*. You can buy passata in the supermarket but make sure it is the real deal and that it does not contain seeds.

Constant Mucus in the Sinuses?
Symptoms caused by lectins only last as long as you continue to ingest the guilty parties. Eating a variety of fruit and veg rather than being a big spinach eater, for example, is one way of reducing the effects of lectins. Fermented plant foods are another way of removing the problem. The creation of mucus can be the bodies defence mechanism to expel lectins.[1] A mucus lining can form in the sinuses as well as on the gut wall and sometimes this can be caused by lectins, especially in milk. Find the culprit and possibly remove that constant trickle at the back of the nose and throat.

The Grain Gamble
As we know gluten is a problematic lectin for many and even gluten free grains are loaded with lectins.[2] Unrefined grains contain more nutrients than refined grain but they also contain more lectins.

In Evolutionary Terms, Grains Are New To Us
Prior to the agricultural age in the Neolithic era beginning 9500BC, grains were only available in small quantities on a seasonal basis. Today the standard western diet is very highly grain based with most meals containing bread, pasta, rice or other cereal crop.

Wholegrains and Insulin
Our shift toward grain consumption has maybe gone too far and this could be having an impact on our on-going battle to minimise insulin resistance. Our grain consumption is, of course, on top of an overly high sugar consumption. Most government guidelines suggest consuming over 300g a day from grains and starchy vegetables, such as potatoes. Apart from not being as nutrient dense as vegetables, what will this level of grain consumption do to our insulin status? *As individuals, responsible for ourselves, we have to make our own decision; which model to pursue …. We're on our own!*

The Comfort They Give
Yet, foods made from grains such as bread have a comfort element to them and some may feel it is too miserable to exist without it. I used to love bread but I no longer have it and no longer miss it.

The Gas They Give!
I certainly no longer miss the immediate bloating and general discomfort I felt after eating bread, pizza or a plate of pasta. Foods with refined grains can feed pathogens (bad bacteria in our gut).

A Little of What You Fancy ….
Instead I enjoy roast potatoes occasionally. Or a bowl of white rice cooked in chicken stock, consumed in moderation and combined within a meal of fibrous vegetables and a little protein and a generous amount of fat. When allowed to cool overnight, both white rice and potatoes gain healthy levels of resistant starch. Rice left longer than that should not really be consumed. The Mediterranean diet often features cold potatoes served with olive oil and herbs or cold rice salads.

Legumes and Anti-Nutrients

Some will argue that legumes should be avoided altogether but nothing is ever that black and white since they are rich in fibre. Yet legumes, like many plant foods, contain the anti-nutrients: phytic acid or phytates as well as lectins.

Phytic acid can bind to certain minerals also contained within the food item and prevent mineral absorption, in particular zinc and iron. It can also interfere with our digestive enzymes.

Protective Processes

Soaking, fermenting, sprouting and pressure-cooking go a long way to resolving lectin issues but most of these traditions have been lost in the west.

A Word of Warning

Lectins are resistant to dry heat. Using white wheat flour alternatives in baking such as chickpea flour, for example, may cause increased irritation.

Are Supermarket Apples Picked Too Soon?

The problem with eating fruit out of season is that it has to travel from afar. Growers and supermarkets may want to pick fruit too early from the trees. Fruits may contain more lectins at an earlier stage in their growing cycle than they would do if they were picked when ripe. Another reason to eat locally grown, seasonal food.

Experiment for yourself

Excluding foods for a period of time is the best way to assess whether certain types of foods affect you or not.

CHAPTER 17: THE SUPER POWERS OF STOCKS AND BROTHS

Chicken Stock And Bone Broth – Cheap and Easy Goodness

Today we tend to buy much of our meat filleted. The routine of making stock out of left over bone and cartilage once common, is now rare.

"We're missing a trick, not making stocks and broths" Whether a child, a young adult rushing around, an elderly person or someone suffering from ill health, homemade stocks and broths offer an incredible source of important goodness in an easy to digest way.

Easy to Make - Versatile to Consume
Full of Goodness - Easy to Digest

What Makes a Good Stock or Broth?

A good broth or stock is an opportunity to incorporate into our diets nutrients that are often, wastefully discarded, in modern eating habits, that can be obtained through the skin, cartilage and bone of animals and that offer health and vitality in a versatile and nutrient dense way. Many of the nutrients on offer in stocks and broths are being purchased at great expense in nutritional supplements.

Even if you don't follow the recipes included here to the letter and you cut corners – the important thing is that you incorporate stocks into your routine. Add them to soups, gravy or absorb it into rice.

Stocks are a big nutritional leap forward for all the family

What Do Stocks And Broths Contain That Are So Good For You?

Calcium, Magnesium, Phosphorous, Potassium, Silicon, Sulphur, Trace Minerals (All sold as expensive supplements). For children and the elderly bone stock offers good levels of both highly absorbable calcium and magnesium to promote bone and dental health amongst other things.

Sulphur Attracts toxic compounds and draws them out of the body. (NB other sulphur containing foods that do this are garlics, onions and cruciferous vegetables.
Cysteine *that forms Glutathione* (Sold as an expensive supplement) Aids the breakdown of mucous in the lungs, a very powerful antioxidant and an important detoxifier that assists in drawing out heavy metals from the body such as cadmium, lead and mercury. Transports nutrients for immune system function
Glycine: (Sold as an expensive supplement). Is found in significantly greater concentrations in skin and bones of animals than in meat. Glycine helps fight inflammation. It has significant effect on mental health, is calming and aids good sleep.
Glucosamine: (Sold as an expensive supplement). Although produced in the body, as we grow older levels can diminish. Stocks and broths offer it and help to maintain healthy joints and cartilage and counteract age related arthritic pain. **Gelatine**: An important characteristic of gelatine is that it draws water towards it, so when used in cooking whether a soup with vegetables or a sauce over meat it enables proper and healthy digestion to occur.
Supports healthy hair and nails.

Healing Leaky Gut A good, 'gloopy' gelatine is formed when stock is slow-cooked for a good few hours. For many who suffer from 'Leaky Gut' it helps to heal the lining of the intestines providing easy to digest nutrients.   This allows the gut a chance to repair itself and stop larger molecules of food crossing the gut wall. This can be the cause of many allergies and immune disorders.

It offers relief also to serious intestinal disorders such as Crohn's disease and colitis. Those suffering these conditions find the gelatine in stocks and broths offer easily digestible protein.

STOCK RECIPES

Chicken Stock Recipe
As ever try to ensure the source of your chicken is the best you can get.
The easiest option is to use the left over carcass of Sunday roast chicken.
Alternatively your butcher may be able to provide you with chicken carcasses if he prepares his own fillets in his shop.
Chicken wings and drumsticks are another option.
The important thing is to include skin, bone and cartilage of the chicken.
Put into a large pot with lid together with:
- 5 litres of water
- 2 tablespoons of vinegar or lemon (this helps to draw out the minerals)
- 1 large onion coarsely chopped
- 2 large carrots coarsely chopped
- 3 celery sticks coarsely chopped
- A handful of unchopped parsley
- Some Bay Leaves
- Sprinkle of Peppercorns

Instructions
- Place your carcass and chicken pieces in pot with the water and vinegar this will begin the leaching process of minerals from the bones.
- Add the vegetables.
- Add the water and vinegar and let stand for an hour.
- Bring to the boil but do not allow to boil too long. This will bring scum to the surface that can then be skimmed off.
- Add herbs and spices you wish to include and leave to simmer with lid on.
- Cook on hob at lowest temperature that allows a very gentle simmer to occur or in the oven if you prefer, at just over 110 degrees ensuring that a gentle simmer is occurring.
- Cook for a minimum of 6 hours and up to 24 hours. The longer, the better the flavour.
- You will not experience the 'gloop' until the stock has been allowed to cool.
- It is best not to leave stocks hanging around at room temperature for too long as this ideal temperature for bugs to breed.

- Once the stock has been removed from heat. Allow to cool slightly and then place pot in a sink half filled with cold water. This will allow the pot to cool slightly faster.
- Strain the stock in a colander removing all meat, bones, vegetables.
- Once cooled either:
1. Place pot in fridge overnight and in the morning you will find that the stock has congealed and formed a layer of fat on top. Skim off the fat. The stock below will be a lovely jelly consistency ready to be divided into containers or ice cube trays and placed in the freezer for storage.
2. Stir fat back in and divide into containers.
3. You can store for several days in the fridge and several months in the freezer.

Bone Stock Recipe

As before try to obtain the best quality source of food that you can.

Variety is important for a healthy bone stock so ask the butcher what he can offer you. Some butcher's prepare bone bags for consumption by pets. Chopped bones where the marrow is exposed is great as it provides a lot of nutrients and flavour. Also include pieces of meat on the bone like rib or neck.

- 1.5 kg of bone with marrow and1 kg of meat on bone eg ribs or neck
- 2 tablespoons of vinegar (this helps to draw out the minerals)
- 1 large onion, 2 large carrots, 3 celery sticks coarsely chopped
  To be added after skimming off of surface scum has occurred:
- A handful of unchopped parsley (some leave this for only the last 10 minutes of cooking time)
- Some Bay Leaves
- Other sprigs of herbs of choice, tied for easy removal later
- Sprinkle of Peppercorns

Instructions

- Place your bones with marrow in pot with the water and vinegar this will begin the leaching process of minerals from the bones.
- Meanwhile roast the bones with meat on them until brown.
- Add the roasted bones to the pot of bones in water and add the vegetables.
- Ensure water level is up to an inch below rim of pot.

- Bring to the boil but do not allow to boil too long. This will bring scum to the surface that can then be skimmed off.
- Add desired herbs and spices and leave to simmer with lid on.
- Cook on hob at lowest temperature that allows a very gentle simmer to occur or in the oven at just over 110 degrees ensuring that it has reached a very gentle simmer.
- Bone stock should ideally cook for a minimum of 12 hours and up to 72 hours. Though in my experience I have reached a lovely gelatinous gloop after just 8 hours!
- You will not experience the 'gloop' until the stock has been allowed to cool.
- It is best not to leave stocks hanging around at room temperature for too long as this ideal temperature for bugs to breed.
- Once the stock has been removed from heat. Allow to cool, slightly and then place pot in a sink half filled with cold water. This will allow the pot to cool slightly faster.
- Strain stock in a colander removing all meat, bones, vegetables and herbs.
- Once cooled place pot in fridge overnight.
- In the morning you will find that the stock has congealed and formed a layer of fat . This can be removed and stored in the fridge for use as fat for cooking. The stock below will be a lovely jelly consistency ready to divide into containers or ice cube trays and placed in the freezer for storage.
- Store stock for several days in the fridge and several months in the freezer.

…. And Don't Forget Fish Stock

In Asia and the Mediterranean the tradition of fish stock is more prevalent. Have you met anyone recently trying to persuade their fishmonger to give them the left over fish heads to make a good stock? Fish stock is rich in minerals including iodine and fish heads contain the benefits of the thyroid gland.

Stocks: Gentle On The Gut, Nurture You Well When You Are Unwell

Stocks and broths are gentle on the digestive system. They are good nutritious ways of taking in more goodness when feeling unwell and off your food. They are especially good for those suffering from digestive and inflammatory issues as they allow the gut to heal but still feed the body.

CHAPTER **18**: ALL DISEASE IS CAUSED BY DEFICIENCY OR TOXICITY

Time To Pay More Attention To The Chemical Assault

Toxicity

We need to pay more attention to products that we buy and use such as cosmetics, domestic cleaning products, fire retardant chemicals and pollution in general that surround us in our modern world. One way or another our bodies' are bombarded with chemicals on a daily basis: inhaled and absorbed into our lungs, ingested or absorbed through our skin.

Are You Prepared to Eat Your Moisturiser?

Should we be adopting the view that "if we are not prepared to eat it then why should we be prepared to put it on our skin?"

We should take stock and think whether all these products are really necessary and whether, maybe, there are some more natural alternatives we could use instead. It might even work out cheaper. Most of us will have thought along these lines at one time or another but the difference today is that our bodies are in danger of reaching a point of 'saturation'. Marketing machines and mass production have been working flat out, and efficiently, for decades and the result is that, without realising it, we have been talked into using so very many products that we didn't even know we needed.

We double glaze our houses, refuse to open our windows
and resort to air fresheners …

Deficiency

A varied, healthy diet of whole foods that have been thoughtfully sourced for quality and freshness is obviously vital for our health but, on my journey, I have gone from resisting the idea of supplementation to believing that we have no choice but to supplement if we wish to preserve our well-being. Depending on who we are, what we do and where we live what we need to supplement can vary substantially. Choosing our vitamins and minerals needs to be done carefully and investigated fully, paying attention to our body's ability to absorb what it consumes, the doses we take, and the origin of the supplements.

The Triage Theory

Definition of 'Triage': the sorting of patients (as in an emergency room) according to the urgency of their need for care.

Bruce Ames, Ph.D, born in 1920 is Professor Emeritus of Biochemistry and Molecular Biology at the University of California Berkeley and at the age of 90 is also senior scientist at the Children's Hospital Oakland Research Institute. Ames believes that we are significantly deficient in approximately 30 different vitamins and minerals and that this will affect our prospects for longevity even if we appear healthy now. He believes that what we require to reduce disease may not be enough to optimize longevity in the long run.

Ames published a paper in 2006 that theorized that when a cell starts running low on certain vitamins, for example, it will carefully allocate what it has to the protein enzymes necessary for immediate survival instead of directing it towards mechanisms responsible for preventing cancers and long-term disease. (Triage) To have a sense of perspective whilst many proteins in the body use vitamins, zinc also, for example, is required by approximately 2000 proteins and magnesium is involved in over 300 internal mechanisms.

"So, what you're doing is trading long-term health for short-term health ... You may look perfectly OK, but if you're not eating a good diet, you're ageing yourself fast."
Bruce Ames

Particular Vitamins & Minerals To Take A Closer Look At

Variation in recommended vitamin supplement dosage is a major subject in itself. For example vitamin C tablets can be found in shops at 500mg when in fact some advocate 6,000-12,000mg (discussed later) and upward a day, spread out over the day. Tablets at 500mg would prove to be a costly way of consuming this high quantity of vitamin C.

I do not believe we can realistically take in all our recommended daily allowance of vitamins and minerals through food alone and in addition, ironically, some of the recommended allowances may be entirely too low.

Look Out For The Vitamins and Minerals That Were Abundant During our Evolution – We Probably Need More

There are certain vitamins and minerals that during our evolution over tens of thousands of years may have been more abundant to us such as magnesium (fourth most common element in the earth) and Vitamin D (abundant through sun exposure). We will have evolved to be fundamentally dependent on these easily accessible nutrients. However the lives we led that caused us to evolve in this way do not match the world we live in today. We do not eat the same foods and we do not necessarily get the same amount of time outdoors and thus we can suffer from fundamental deficiencies.

On my journey of discovery I have come across a few vitamins and mineral facts that really stood out. Obviously all the vitamins and minerals, including trace minerals are important to us but the following have been particularly interesting.

Magnesium – Vitamin D – Vitamin K2 – Vitamin C

Magnesium

Magnesium is a vital mineral to our bodies involved in over 300 metabolic functions and essential for maintaining balanced muscle and nerve function. It is important for healthy bones, steady heart rhythm, stable blood pressure and healthy heart.

If the average person was eating well and consuming a plentiful, daily serving of dark leafy greens, dark chocolate, fish and avocados for example, then they would probably be getting sufficient levels of this mineral. Much is said about soil depletion causing lack of magnesium but remember that chlorophyll is what gives a vegetable its green colour and chlorophyll cannot form without magnesium.

Reasons For Deficiency

Unfortunately many of us do not get enough in our diet. In addition, the sugars and carbohydrates we eat use up our magnesium store as it is needed in significant quantity just simply to metabolise the sugar laden foods we eat.

The situation is the same with chemicals and toxins that enter our body. Here too magnesium is necessary to enable our body to deal with the toxins. For these reasons many of us are severely lacking in this most important mineral to carry out its functions that enable our bodies to work efficiently.

If supplementation is favoured the issue of toxicity is not a problem as excess consumption of magnesium is regulated by the body and excreted. (Beware, this is not the case with calcium that is stored by the body and could build to unwelcome levels if supplemented).

Deficiency Can Be Very Serious
One of the signs of magnesium deficiency is muscle spasm, a common example is foot or calf cramp typically experienced when in bed especially when stretching but muscle spasm can manifest itself in far more serious ways.

Muscle spasms associated with the arteries and the heart can lead to heart attack and strokes. Sudden death in athletes can be brought on by excess sweating and loss of minerals exacerbated by consumption of sweetened sports drinks that both lead to severe magnesium depletion. Magnesium deficiency is common and can lead to constriction of the arteries leading to high blood pressure.

Back Pain
A lot of back pain can be attributed to lack of magnesium. The tightening of the very many muscles in our backs from the neck to the lumbago could be addressed with the reduction of sugars and carbohydrates and the replenishing of magnesium levels. Traditional knowledge would have encouraged bathing in Epsom Salts, for their magnesium content and the mineral's absorbability through the skin.

Effect on Other Essential Nutrients
Lack of magnesium will hamper other essential nutrients to carry out their function properly as they require to work in synergy to serve their purposes.

The Magnesium – Calcium Relationship Is Important
Many people, especially women over a certain age are encouraged to supplement their calcium intake but without a proper balance of magnesium it can lead to an increased risk of heart attack, osteoporosis, kidney stones and other issues. [1] Magnesium aids muscle relaxation and calcium aids muscle contraction. When calcium is supplemented and not balanced with magnesium then muscles (including your heart) can be at risk of going into spasm (heart attack).

In addition to this calcium on its own cannot be assimilated into the bone. It needs to team up with magnesium, Vitamin D and Vitamin K2 (that in turn require other vitamins and minerals to function efficiently). Instead calcium can create calcification in the soft tissue causing hardening of the arteries. (1)

Again these relationships are described in simple terms but highlight just why it is so important to eat well and have a good variety of food to maximise your chances of taking in your vitamins and minerals. It also emphasizes why the need for doctors to understand nutrition is so important.

Vitamin C
This vitamin is so important that it is produced in nearly all living organisms both plant and animal. Unfortunately humans lost this ability millions of years ago.
The scientist Irwin Stone said of this event:
".... (it) may be eventually regarded as the greatest single physiological and biochemical catastrophe to have happened to Man in the course of evolution" (2)

Vitamin C (also known as ascorbic acid) is a powerful antioxidant. It fights infection and free radicals. It helps us maintain healthy skin, bones, teeth, and blood cells and digestion. It is what keeps us standing as it is vital for the production of collagen that heals our soft tissue and gives it its elasticity.

We are familiar with vitamin C deficiency due to the plight of sailors up until the 1770s who suffered from scurvy on their long sea voyages with no access to the vitamin in their food. Their suffering was characterised by bleeding gums, nose bleeds, rupturing of capillaries and thus bruising and frequent infection.

Today we are told that the RDA (recommended daily allowance) for vitamin C is 90mg. It may be the case though that such a small amount is only enough to prevent the outward signs of scurvy. We may, however, still be significantly deficient in vitamin C to be suffering from the symptoms of scurvy at a sub-clinical level. In other words we may be suffering health problems due to this deficiency but not attributing it to the right cause.

The Question of "Mega-dosing"

Listening to recordings made by Linus Pauling, a winner of two Nobel Peace Prizes for science and famously the author of "Vitamin C and the Common Cold" I was taken with his explanation of how deficiency of ascorbic acid reduced the elasticity of our arteries and was a major cause for the lesions or small tears in our arteries that can lead us down the path to eventual arterial blockages, strokes and heart attacks. Linus Pauling advocated taking much higher doses of the vitamin, pointing out that the vast majority of animals produce their own vitamin C and increase this production at moments of stress, injury, illness and trauma. These things together with pollution use up vitamin C and in humans we are left lacking.

Due to a genetic mutation we lost a vital enzyme that animals use to release ascorbic acid in to their bloodstream as and when required. Unlike other species that also suffered this mutation and died out quickly we survived due to the fact that in jungle areas we had vitamin c-rich food all year round.

According to The Vitamin C Foundation 1997:

"The fact that almost all species continue to make vitamin C suggests that the amount of this vitamin generally available from diet is not enough for optimum nutrition except in exceptional circumstances such as a tropical environment."

".... Under normal circumstances the daily amount produced (in animals), adjusted for comparison to a 70 kg man, is somewhere between 3,000 mg and 15,000 mg, with an average of 5,400 mg."

"More than 50% of people require over 2,500 mg (of ascorbic acid) to reach maximum absorption. "

"Vitamin C is one of the least toxic substances known to man".

Linus Pauling took high levels of Vitamin C, staggered throughout the day. He lived to 93 mentally and physically agile.

Vitamin D

No Sunshine in the On-Line World

Vitamin D is known as the sunshine vitamin. It is fundamental to health.
Offices, computers, electronic distractions, TV, texting, in other words the 'on-line' world is keeping us indoors and away from the sunshine.

Direct exposure to sunlight is the most efficient way to maximise our vitamin D levels. For those of us not lucky enough to live in the Tropics but in countries where the winters are longer and on top of that those of us that "do not work in the fields" but work indoors, exposure to the sun is fairly limited. In addition to this, today, when we do go outdoors we are encouraged to cover up or wear high protection sunscreen.

Science is busy looking at the whole issue of Vitamin D at the moment and there is an awareness that our fear of exposure to sunlight due to skin cancer needs to be balanced with need for Vitamin D as its deficiency in our bodies is causing many problems.

Vitamin D is fundamentally important for cellular health, helping to prevent certain cancers, including skin cancers! (3) It is required for immunity, bone and muscle function, mood, depression, insomnia, organ and brain health…. Well that's about everything really!

Go Slightly Pink But Don't Burn
According to the Vitamin D Council:
"The two main ways to get vitamin D are by exposing your bare skin to sunlight and by taking vitamin D supplements. You can't get the right amount of vitamin D your body needs from food. The most natural way to get vitamin D is by exposing your bare skin to sunlight (ultraviolet B rays)."

Depending on who we are, where we live and what we do, we are all bound to have very different levels of Vitamin D. It may be the case that testing our Vitamin D levels is an important step forward in preventative care and correct and supervised supplementation could have an important impact on our health. In my quest for reason and balance and as far as the sun is concerned my preference is to sit out in the sun whenever the opportunity occurs usually for about 30 minutes until there is slight pinkness and then cover up to avoid burning.

Things Are Never Simple
How much vitamin D your body actually makes depends on a number of factors:

The angle of the sun
- Where you are in the world (on the Equator or Northern Europe)
- Whether it is winter, summer, spring or autumn
- What time of day it is, with the midday sun obviously offering the strongest rays

Your ethnic grouping
- Those, say of Indian or African descent with darker skins are more susceptible to deficiency in Vitamin D living in northern climates compared to fairer skinned individuals.
- For darker skinned individuals more exposure to the sun is required to gain adequate amounts of the vitamin.

Altitude
- Are you up a mountain where the rays are stronger

Your Age
- With age the less able is the body to make vitamin D from the sun

Skin Exposure
- Are you in a burqa or a bikini!

Vitamin D Council Recommended Intake For Vitamin D in International Units (IU)
Infants and Children: 1000IU – 2000IU maximum
Adults: 5000IU – 10,000IU maximum
To put these recommendations into context your body can produce 10,000-25,000IU Vitamin D after just a short time of full body sun exposure. Vitamin D is fat-soluble and supplements should be consumed with meals with fat of some sort.

Vitamin K2

Most people and even some doctors have never heard of Vitamin K2. Vitamin K1 the blood-clotting vitamin was discovered in 1929 by a German scientist and its letter comes from Koagulations vitamin. The two K vitamins are very different. K1 is found in plant foods and K2 is found in animal sources and fermented foods. There is much excitement surrounding Vitamin K2. It has largely gone un-noticed and much more research needs to take place and clinical evidence gathered but the growing belief today is that:

Vitamin K2 plays a crucial role in directing calcium to bones and teeth in synergy with Vitamin D. Importantly, it also prevents the build up of calcium in soft tissue (calcification) such as the arteries that can lead to arterial plaque leading to strokes and heart attacks.

In the past the higher prevalence of fermented foods would have meant more intake of Vitamin K2. Today supplementation is being advised by some for its strong association with possible reduction in heart disease. (4)

CHAPTER 19: STRESS, BABOONS AND BRITISH CIVIL SERVANTS

We all keep being told that stress is bad but we do not really take the fact on board. On my journey of discovery I have read quite a lot about stress but the message never really sank in until I found a National Geographic/Stanford University documentary on the work of Stanford University, Neurobiologist Robert Sapolsky and also of Sir Michael Marmot Professor of Epidemiology and Public Health at University College London. (1)

These two individuals were carrying out similar studies in totally different parts of the world. Sapolsky was carrying out a study on the effect of social stress on baboons in Africa. Professor Marmot meanwhile was looking at the social stress of British civil servants.

It transpires that baboons, apart from having to focus on eating for 3 hours a day in order to get their required calories, do not have to worry about anything very much. Not having much to do, however, is pretty bad news. The community of baboons that Sapolsky studied spent most of their spare time "bothering" each other. A lot of tortuous, bullying behaviour took place and depending on where the baboons were in the social pecking order resulted in different levels stress being experienced.

Needless to say the alpha males at the top of the pecking order were doing a lot of the bullying but not receiving anything back. They were in control of their situation and experienced no stress. The baboons lower down the pecking order never knew what to expect next …. From being pounced on, to having their hair pulled to worse – they were constantly in a heightened state of awareness and felt little control over their own situation.

What Sapolsky went on to discover, was really quite shocking. He carried out tests on his community of baboons and looked closely at the state of their arteries. The relationship between position in the hierarchy and narrowing of the arteries due to atherosclerosis was consistent. Those in the top echelons were fit and well and had clear, healthy arteries. As you moved down the social scale the level of "clogging" of the arteries increased and in addition weight also became an issue.

Even more concerning was that when they did comparative studies of the primates' brains, further data came out to support the social strata theory. Brain atrophy (shrinkage) was also apparent leading to reduction in the cognitive behaviour of those primates lower down the social ladder.

Baboons Don't Smoke
The beauty of the study on baboons was that it was able to remove certain factors that might muddy the waters when looking at effects of stress on the human body. Baboons do not drink alcohol, they do not smoke and they all eat, pretty much, the same diet.

Perceived Control Over Your Existence Is Important
Professor Marmot's study that had spanned 40 years, looking at 28,000 British civil servants came to similar conclusions.

The British civil service has a very rigid hierarchical employment ranking system. Again, like in the baboon community the civil servants at the top felt much more in control over their existence than those at the bottom. Being able to observe so many people over such a time period, individuals who would have similar health care benefits and education, was very valuable. Marmot observed that ranking "intimately related to risk of disease and length of life".

Whatever your view is on this research the main thing to take away is that stress …. is really bad and should be managed as much as possible. The perceived and unperceived physiological impact it has on our body cannot be underestimated. Stress will make you want to eat, hungry or not. Eating the wrong foods will only heighten anxiety and make the situation worse, whilst the right foods will minimise negative feelings.

Always remember exercise is a good stress reliever.

CHAPTER 20:   SLEEP AND EXERCISE - POWER TOOLS FOR HEALTH

Sleep
Whatever we do, we must be sure to nurture and protect good quality sleep at night. Eight hours seems to be considered optimal. When we sleep our body:
- Rests
- Protects our hormone function
- Enhances our immunity
- Is rebalancing brain chemicals
- Keeps our hunger in check
- Heals
- Stores our memories
- Is busy repairing blood vessels
- Is eliminating toxins

Or in other words, if we don't sleep well, none of these vital protective functions can be carried out properly and we severely increase our risk of ill health. We must find the resolve to remove all electronics not only from our bedrooms but especially, if we are to do our duty and protect them, from our childrens' bedrooms. Even if they are protected from the cyber world, sleep disruption will affect everyone who is using these gadgets. Effectively firing up the brain just before closing our eyes to try to go to sleep.

The Power Of Exercise
Regular exercise is absolutely fundamental to maintaining health, especially resistance training. In addition and notably aerobic exercise has the power to stimulate the growth of new brain cells a process called neurogenesis. In addition memory is enhanced by regular, short sessions of exercise that raise your heartbeat.

Exercise helps combat chronic inflammation thus helping to ward off disease. As always though, in the pursuit of reason and balance, keep an eye on 'wear and tear'. Pounding the pavements on a regular basis may be good for your heart but what effect will it have on your knee joints in the long-term? Ensure that you vary your exercise and avoid repetitive movements that impact your joints. With antibiotic resistance becoming more prevalent, in the future hip and knee joint operations may not be so run of the mill as they are today…. So look after them!

CHAPTER 21:   SO WHAT IS BALANCED EATING?

What Is The Most Important Thing We Have To Balance in Our Diet?

In trying to answer this question, at an extremely fundamental level, one of the things that comes to mind is the fact that, in laboratory experiments, calorie restricted mice live longer than non-calorie restricted mice. We have certainly suffered from calorie overload, with our western way of eating and perhaps we have suffered from this for thousands of years since the advent of farming and the growing of crops and the use of grains.

The Nation's Lunchtime Staple

Just think of how often and easy it is to overload with empty calories, a fizzy, canned drink, with a petrol station sandwich, a packet of crisps and a chocolate bar. No wonder there is trouble.

As the chapter title points out, though, calorie restriction needs to be balanced ... with what? - Emphasis on nutrient density. When we do put something in our mouth it should be rich in the nutrients that enable us to thrive. The healthy fats and proteins that are the materials our body is made of. The vitamins including the fat soluble vitamins, the minerals, the essential fatty acids such as Omega 3 and 6, the antioxidants and polyphenols in plant foods and the fibre to feed our gut bugs.

If we eat healthy foods that do not create the hormone imbalances that lead to cravings, then we should rediscover the fine art of eating when we are hungry and stopping when we are full. This balance is aided and maintained by good sleep, reducing stress and being active, busy, sociable and generous in spirit.

Jokers in the Pack

Yet there is not a 'one size fits all'. Apart from anything else our gut bacteria are like jokers in the pack. They have enormous impact; their ability to change at speed, depending on what, we eat makes them elusive and complex for science to understand. We are learning, slowly, how different gut bacterial profiles in different people can completely alter their response to different types of food and how variety in the diet is beneficial. The profile of the bacterial cultures in our gut should alter seasonally, in accordance with the food that is available to us.

Avoid Entrenching into Extreme Ways of Eating

So we must adopt a pragmatic view based on knowledge, observation and common sense. Once we have dispensed with sugar we can reconnect with our own bodies and be more receptive to the signals it gives us. We must self-experiment, because what works for one person may not work for another. Nonetheless, more understanding of how our body works is key.

The Displacement of Traditional Ways of Eating

The following list may act as a gentle reminder of the changes that have taken place in the way we eat. Weston Price (1870-1948) was an American dentist who travelled the world identifying healthy cultures and peoples based on their dental health. He sought the factors responsible for healthy, straight teeth within a broad palate mouth. He found those factors among isolated, non-industrial communities. Weston Price highlighted the following:

Traditional Foods Among Isolated, Non-Industrial Communities	"Displacing Foods of Modern Commerce"
Traditional foods varied widely	Increased emphasis on carbs through:
Large and small, land and sea animals	White flour
All animal material consumed including fat, organs, bone and skin	White sugar
Eggs, Dairy products including butter fat	White rice
Whole cereals	Syrups, jams
Tubers, Fruit and vegetables	Canned goods
Coconut	Vegetable oils

(1)

Fat and Protein: The Building Blocks of Our Body

It is worth noting that 65% of the calories
of these traditional communities
came from animal food.(1)

Fat and protein are the only foods that provide the building blocks for our body. They are nutrient dense and help maintain a feeling of fullness for longer compared to carbohydrates. Meat, eggs, dairy and seafood provide more protein, and nutrition gramme per gramme than beans, legumes or other plant sources.

If we choose to eat meat then we must aim to buy quality meat that is derived from animals that have been reared and fed healthily, in harmony with the environment, and for this we must be prepared to pay.

Animal Fat
Animal fat, especially, gives flavour to food and where previously it was removed it had to be substituted with sugar to make the food palatable.

Polyunsaturated vegetable oils have been promoted heavily, to replace saturated fat, over the last several decades and as we have seen in Chapter 8 this has been, in many cases, a wholly toxic substitute for us.

The highly rated, traditional Mediterranean diet used large amounts of monounsaturated fat from olive oil and also ample amounts of fish so omega 3 fat was prominent in the diet. The people of the Mediterranean did not, traditionally, shy away from animal fat, using far more of the animal than we do today. Polyunsaturated fat did not feature significantly at all.

Have We Been Vastly Underestimating the Importance of Quality Animal Fat?
Quality fat should be reintroduced much more liberally into the diet as long as carbohydrate content is lowered. Remember high carbohydrate and high fat are the *worst* possible combination. Put polyphenol rich, quality olive oil on salads or butter from pasture raised cows on steamed vegetables.

Fatty cuts of quality meat, animal fat and oily fish in general are the best sources of the fat-soluble vitamins A, D3, E and K, together with choline and essential fatty acids. It is worth noting that animal fat allows better absorption of fat soluble vitamins eaten at the same time in other foods. In addition the more fat consumed in a meal, the greater the absorption of the fat soluble vitamins.[1] Weston Price noted in his travels that the common factor in isolated, non-industrialised communities displaying excellent overall health was their levels of fat-soluble vitamin intake based on dietary focus on fish, seafood, eggs, dairy and animal fat.

Animal Protein

We should not underestimate the nutritional density of animal and fish protein including eggs and dairy: Vitamin A (in Retinol form is only available in animal products), Omega 3 in oily fish (does not require conversion in the body compared to plant based sources). B12 is only obtainable in animal products. Plus vitamins D3 and K2 and more concentrated amounts of minerals are only available in a varied meat and fish diet.

Deficiency in vitamins D3 and K2 is common in society at large today, causing, in particular, calcification and hardening of the arteries. Vitamin A (Retinol) deficiency is also causing health issues, most of which will not be consciously linked and therefore not attributed to deficiency in this vitamin; however, we may see, in the future, more focus on Vitamin A (Retinol) in the same way as we have seen increased interest in Vitamin D3 in mainstream medicine.

Grains and Vegetables

Grain-based foods, compared to vegetables, are less nutritious lacking the overall combination of fibre, polyphenols, antioxidants, vitamins and minerals that vegetables provide. Grains will stimulate higher levels of insulin compared to most vegetables. The energy lost from eating less bread, rice and pasta should be replaced with, insulin sparing, healthy fats.

THE DIRECTIONS WE HAVE TAKEN TO TRY AND IMPROVE OUR HEALTH:

1. Veganism - Not A Way Of Eating That Should Be Embarked On Lightly

It is not good enough to just eat vegan food. It is difficult (many say impossible), with this way of eating, to get the healthy fats and proteins in the quantities required to maintain long-term health. If Bruce Ames' Triage Theory is correct, vegans may not discover this until it is too late. If veganism is to be pursued, it needs to be done in an extremely well informed way. Yet, ultimately, we are guaranteed better levels of nutrition when benefitting from the concentration of fats, proteins, minerals and vitamins in a piece of meat or fish. Veganism is popular and promoted to the young. Are teenagers, who are still growing and who may lead erratic lifestyles, really going to achieve good health if they pursue this way of eating?

Vegetable oils do not provide vitamins A, D3, E and K as are found in animal fats. In addition the levels of polyunsaturated omega 6 found in vegetable oils can be highly inflammatory for the body as highlighted in Chapter 8. Omega 3 and vitamin A from plant sources are not as efficient, beneficial or even obtainable (in the case of vitamin B12) when compared to animal/fish sources of these nutrients.

With questionable farming methods, including the use of pesticides and increasing soil poverty, many vegans will find it difficult to obtain sufficient nutrient concentrations in today's well-travelled plant foods.

2. Vegetarianism Makes Life Easier

Again, those that pursue it need to be more focused on food and eating well to compensate for the lack of meat or fish. As with vegans, the fact that the nutrients in our soil are not necessarily as abundant as they once were, together with plant foods clocking up many air miles, it is probably more important to take additional vitamins and minerals in supplement form. Eggs and butter from grass fed beef will be very valuable to vegetarians for the fat soluble vitamins A, D3, E and K. (Sorry did I mention fat soluble vitamins again!) Vegetarians are likely to consume more beneficial fermentable fibres that feed our good gut bacteria, which form the basis of our immune system, compared to meat eaters. Plant foods need to be varied and lectin build up needs to be avoided to prevent possible gut irritation. The consumption of grains should also be tempered by an awareness of insulin stimulation.

3. Palaeolithic Diet: Eating Like Our Hunter-Gatherer Ancestors

This approach adopts our Palaeolithic forefathers' ways of feeding before the advent of agriculture and the growing of crops. Focus is maintained on meat, especially highly nutritious organ meats, fat and seafood. Only plant food that was available to pick was consumed, such as fermentable fibre-rich tubers and vegetation and fruit.

The West has turned away from the traditional use of all parts of the animal favouring, nutritionally less valuable, pre-packaged, filleted, lean meat from supermarkets, rather than the full range of cuts and organs available from a traditional butcher. Today, if you want to shop in a supermarket you will be hard pressed to get hold of bones, fish heads and off-cuts to make a good stock. Many in the Paleo community follow a ketogenic way of eating and have adopted intermittent fasting.

4. The Ketogenic Diet: Beware of *Unhealthy* Fats

We have covered this way of eating earlier in the book and looked at the benefits gained from becoming metabolically flexible, easily switching from burning sugars to burning fats to fuel our body.

As achieving ketosis requires consumption of less carbohydrates and a higher consumption of fat, it is important to understand the difference between healthy and unhealthy fats.

Those that pursue a ketogenic diet should perhaps take care not to allow the consumption of healthy fibre to slip, especially resistant starches.

5. Intermittent Fasting and an Eye on Nutrient Dense Food

For all those committed to a desire to pursue intermittent fasting to varying degrees they should be equally committed to ensuring that all calorie intake is as nutrient dense and beneficial as possible. It is important to ensure that salt levels (electrolytes) do not go down too low, particularly sodium, potassium and magnesium.

6. Caloric Restriction/Fasting Mimicking Diet

Dr Valter Longo has been a prominent researcher in this area. His experiments have highlighted how periods of time fasting and then re-feeding, has led to some very positive effects on inflammatory and autoimmune conditions. Emphasis should be placed on the fact that the improvements are seen during the re-feeding phase of the fasting cycle. A report that came out, of his work, in 'Cell' in June 2016[1a] highlighted that his fasting mimicking diet helped to:

- Reduce inflammation
- Suppress autoimmunity (where the immune system turns on the body and attacks it – the basis of autoimmune diseases)

- "Promote a safe, feasible and effective treatment for Multiple Sclerosis patients."(See also the work of Dr Terry Wahls who recovered dramatically from MS). (2)

7. The Carnivore Diet: The Jury is Out on Long-Term Benefits But It May Be Therapeutic in the Short Term Especially to Those with Gut Issues

As yet there are no long-term studies of the carnivore diet. One concern is what effect the absence of fibre in the diet will have on individuals that pursue this way of eating. In addition there are those that simply eat muscle meat (steaks, etc), whilst others are keen to benefit from the concentrated nutrients in organ meat. Either way the quality of meat consumed will depend entirely on the health and feed that the animal experienced in its life.

Quality meat consumption is beneficial in growing children and those of reproductive age when cell division is important for growth. This process is enabled both by a protein in our body called IGF1 and aided by the consumption of meat. In mid-life when we are still producing elevated levels of IGF1, that promotes cell division, the addition of too much protein may raise our risk of cell proliferation of possible cancerous cells in our body. So from the ages of 50-65 it may be beneficial to reduce levels of meat intake to aid longevity. Production of IGF 1 subsides over the age of about 65, this can lead to muscle loss and frailty. Increased consumption of animal protein, at this age, can help optimize health span and longevity. Dr Valter Longo of the University of Southern California has been a major researcher in this area. (3)

Inflammatory Bowel Disease and the Carnivore Diet

There have been more and more anecdotal indications coming through on-line that seem to show that those with inflammatory bowel conditions benefit from a period of time on a meat-only diet. Why should this be?

Meat is digested higher up in the gut and most of its constituent parts are used by the body for structure and repair. By the time it reaches the colon there is little left to aggravate or cause further inflammation. In addition, it is possible that this way of eating acts as an extreme "removal diet". In other words, this diet suddenly removes ALL plant foods. As we know, many plant foods contain different lectins that can cause inflammatory flare-ups that individuals may not have identified, such as from legumes, pulses or various nightshade vegetables. So, this removal of plant foods and fibre allows the large intestine a total rest whilst allowing the body to maintain a nutrient dense intake of food, through meat. This may be a useful tool for people suffering from diverticulitis, Crohns or colitis, especially in the elderly, who are particularly at risk from malnutrition.

It Wasn't That Long Ago We Were Advised To Eat Less Fat And More Grains
As we have seen there is great division over whole grains but there are a growing number of researchers who believe that when advice changed in the middle of the 20th century to consume less fat, the increased emphasis on grains led to many health problems, caused by the cumulative effect on insulin and the impact of gluten in wheat. A prominent researcher on gluten, is Alessio Fasano, Director of the Mucosal Immunology and Biology Research Centre in Massachusetts. Fasano's research is showing that gluten increases the risk of autoimmune disease for those with a genetic predisposition and not just in those who are gluten intolerant. (4)

Grains May Prevent Us From Living To Our Full Potential in Terms of Quality and Quantity of Life
We certainly did not evolve to eat grains. We have been around for tens of thousands of years yet farming cereal crops only began some 14,000 years ago. Over time, however, grains have become a staple; they have been thoroughly convenient for us as they are inexpensive, easy and have a longer shelf life.

We Must Always Accept That Our Ideas Will Be Challenged
As I said right at the beginning of the book we must always be prepared to have our ideas challenged. Gut bacteria and the microbiota is an area where we are barely scratching the surface and the fact that communities live successfully on totally contrasting ways of eating shows how we must keep an open mind on many things. The bacterial world is incredibly adaptable and there are many things we are yet to learn. Notably there are two groups of people who have challenged the world of nutrition and are often cited. They are good case studies to bear in mind:

The Kitavan Paradox

The Kitavans of Papua New Guinea have very low rates of heart disease or cancer despite being consumers of *high levels* of

- unprocessed carbohydrates
- meat
- fish
- saturated fat from coconut
- … and big smokers

What is their secret?

- No processed food
- No wheat
- No refined sugar
- Low iron levels
- Lots of sun exposure
- Low stress
- Fresh and extremely nutritious whole foods
- A good omega3 to 6 ratio
- And lastly a genetic combination that allows the Kitavans to maintain excellent insulin status.

The Inuit Paradox

The Inuit of Greenland on the other hand have, historically, had low heart disease and cancer on a diet high in protein and fat with no fruit or vegetables. They consumed *high levels* of:

- whale meat
- seal meat
- blubber
- organ meats
- wild game

Their secrets were:

- high vitamin and mineral levels
- Animals create their own vitamin C and this was available to the Inuit when consuming animal food, particularly the organ meat.
- High levels of Selenium and
- High levels of Vitamin D

- A healthy Omega 3 to 6 ratio and
- A late winter challenge to avoid starvation advantageously allowed their bodies "a good clear out and repair" in the form of autophagy.

What Do I Eat to Stay Ship-Shape and Sharp?

Personally, I am enjoying food more than ever and what I eat has never been tastier, thanks to a renewed focus on herbs, spices and animal fat, that add flavour to my vegetables, meat, fish and seafood.

Whole grains hardly feature as I wish to maintain a good, on-going insulin status. Also, I am able to consume plenty of fibre from vegetables that are more nutrient dense and often more fibre-rich than whole grains.

Meat and fish remain important but there is a fine line between too much meat and too little that can lead to poorer nutrient levels. So, meat and fish are small side servings (equivalent to a deck of cards) on my plate of vegetables. Topped with a good helping of healthy fats to ensure that I can absorb all those lovely fat-soluble vitamins, keep my body in shape, burning fat for fuel and providing me with those lovely ketones that keep my brain sharp. I eat avocadoes, cheese (particularly unpasteurised), cream and eggs (mother nature's multi-vitamin). I always have bone broth or chicken stock available in my freezer and I make fermented sauerkraut from red cabbage, dill and fennel seeds (my favourite, at the moment, and lovely to eat with cheese).

A couple of days a week, mostly at the weekend, when I am less busy, I increase carbohydrate intake. I look at this as feasting with the family, though it is no longer feasting as I used to know it. I have evolved over time to enjoy different foods and in smaller quantities. It is no hardship nor do I feel I am missing out.

Now that I have my hormones under control, I no longer have cravings, hunger pangs, *nor do I fail to feel full* after eating. There is only so much I can eat in a day. I want to make sure that it is as nutrient dense and fibre packed as possible. So, I would rather eat a moderate amount of quality meat or fish, healthy fats, and nutritious and healthy vegetables, and occasionally a little fruit.

Experiencing Proper Satiety …
Reintroducing proper amounts of healthy, quality fats into a low carbohydrate diet enables one to eat plenty of nutritious and tasty food until a feeling of fullness is achieved … *until proper satiety is felt*. For when satiety is achieved people can go through longer periods of time without eating thus achieving the benefits of longer periods of fasting whilst feeling mentally and physically "on top of the world".

Must We Make Ourselves Ill to Save the Planet Or is There Another Way?
"The EAT-Lancet Commission on Food, Planet & Health", brought together more than 30 'world-leading' scientists from across the globe. In collaboration with *The Lancet,* a weekly peer-reviewed general medical journal, the aim was to reach a scientific consensus defining a healthy and sustainable diet. The Lancet is among the world's oldest, most prestigious, and best-known general medical journals.

The EAT-Lancet Diet was launched in January 2019 and, being well funded will be heavily promoted, moving forward, by a series of global PR events. The document was developed, by 19 commissioners and 18 co-authors from 16 countries, over a period of 3 years.

So What Do They Recommend?
> *The EAT-Lancet diet recommends that meat consumption (including dairy)*
> *be reduced in the developed world by 80%.*

Their recommendation for an adult male would require only 35% of calories to come from fat (100g), 14% of calories to come from protein (90g) and 51% of calories to come from carbohydrates (329g). Thus, for the average man:
- 232g/day of whole grains such as bread and rice
- 50g/day of starchy vegetables
- 300g/day of vegetables and
- 200g/day of fruit
- 100g/day of fat
- 90g/day of protein

Where does a recommendation of 329g/day of carbohydrates leave us in terms of maintaining a healthy insulin status? A comparison of the ratios of macro-nutrients (as a percentage of total calories) from the EAT Lancet and Ketogenic diets are worlds apart. Obviously gramme weights will vary depending on total calories consumed, but the recommendations could not be more polarised:

EAT Lancet recommendations:

Fat	Protein	Carbohydrate
35%	14%	51%

Compared to a Ketogenic diet of:

60%	15-20%	15-20%

Dr Zoe Harcombe reviewed the nutrient value of the EAT-Lancet diet and has concluded that it is nutritionally deficient in B12, vitamins D3 and K2, calcium, iron, potassium and sodium. Additionally, it is deficient in anti-inflammatory Omega 3 that is best sourced from oily fish whilst at the same time is too high in pro-inflammatory Omega 6. Dr Harcombe's full response is detailed and can be viewed on her website: zoeharcombe.com.

We Must Rely On Human Ingenuity Not Compromising Our Health In Order to Secure The Health Of The Planet

On a global scale, moving away from grains is environmentally problematic as it is the most cost effective source of caloric energy both for us and for livestock. Yet this has been shown to have significant consequences on our health and that of animals fed this way. On the other hand we should not pressure people to avoid animal foods as we evolved to be omnivores. In addition it is vital that farming should contain a balance between growing plant foods and rearing livestock as ruminants are essential for maintaining the quality of our soil.

Food wastage must be addressed, and in addition, not wanting to sound flippant, but the west is suffering from consuming a huge energy overload that is making us ill. If we all adopt the concept of fasting, eating less frequently then surely we can focus on growing and consuming less food but better quality food.

So we must be ambitious, positive and push forward, and not underestimate the resourcefulness and ingenuity of our fellow humans to find solutions to these problems. In order to do this we must allow science to seek truth and constantly question 'knowledge'.

CHAPTER 22:   FINAL REFLECTIONS

Diversity And Moderation
These two words sum up, in a nutshell, what is good for us but many people's diets no longer reflect either of these characteristics.

Even those who are keen to eat healthily may tend to fixate on certain things. For example don't eat spinach everyday; instead, focus on a variety of different greens and salads. Add variety and interest to such plates with items such as garlic, onions, eggs, seeds, herbs, spices, other vegetables, pre and probiotic foods, etc.

Try also to alternate the sources of your food i.e. don't necessarily always buy your broccoli from the same place and, as much as possible, eat seasonal and local food.

Reason And Balance
An approach of reason and balance is essential when it comes to health and nutrition; remembering always that our body works holistically and not as independent organs and systems.

Medicine, A Science Of Separate Parts?
We have tended to look at the subject of the body and human health in pockets. Doctors specialise in organs or specific areas of the body. Yet we can see that a more holistic approach is necessary as the body is so inter-connected.

For example, mental conditions are now recognised to be intricately associated with the state of the gut. How often does a psychologist question or suggest to a patient to simultaneously seek advice on their intestinal health as part of a treatment process?

In the same way, much of the research on vitamins has been conducted in isolation of one another. However, all our essential vitamins and minerals work closely together and need each other in order to carry out their beneficial function.

The Risk To Our Health From So Many Medications That Rob Our Nutrients

*"The art of medicine consists in amusing the patient
whilst nature cures the disease"* Voltaire

"Nutrition is the Medicine of the Future"
Twice Nobel Prize Winner Linus Pauling

The incredibly complex inter relationship of nutrients in foods, in our bodies, begs the question, how can we be happy to take as much medication as we do? How can we possibly know what knock on effects the prescriptions we take really have on our bodies or the biochemical chaos they can create within us?

We are encouraged to take too much medication. Older generations may have reminded us to dress warmly, wear a hat, have some broth and an early night if we were at a low ebb. They were the generation who remembered a time before antibiotics and fever-lowering medication, when getting run down or catching a chill could become a little more serious.... We rely on our meds so we do not take care, but we use them liberally at our peril.

By being so ready to resort to medication we can expose ourselves to side effects that can often lead to worse conditions than those initially treated. For example many basic medications can have serious long-term impact on our intestine, damaging the fine balance of beneficial bacteria that we are now discovering plays such an important part in protecting our health in the first place.

In addition our valuable nutrients are taken up to metabolise these drugs adding further to our nutrient deficiencies. Thus our medications can create further problems whilst only patching symptoms and offering no cure.

Heartburn and Acid Reflux
This is a controversial example where a condition is treated with medication that only eases the symptoms. The medication, in fact, goes on to perpetuate the initial condition thus continuing the need for the medication. [1]

In summary the theory works as follows:
- Our lifestyle is such that we, perhaps, eat bigger portions than we ought to. So then we feel overly full.
- We slump on the sofa with a full stomach.
- The pressure of the food in the stomach causes some of the stomach contents (including some stomach acid) to be pushed up into the oesophagus where the lining is too sensitive to withstand the hydrochloric acid from the stomach.
- Heartburn ensues.
- Antacid medications are then taken to neutralise the acid in the stomach to stop it burning when it comes back up into the oesophagus again.
- BUT THEN …. The acidity in the stomach is reduced. This prevents food from being sufficiently broken down and, at the same time, allows bad bugs (that prefer a less acid environment) to multiply in the stomach.
- These bugs go on to feed off the undigested food thus allowing them to multiply further.
- The bi-product of their feeding is gas that accumulates in the stomach and produces bloating.
- The bloating causes pressure in the stomach that leads to more acidity being pushed up into the oesophagus causing more heartburn.
- Leading to the need for more anti acids…
- So, the anti acids alleviate the discomfort but aggravate the overall condition that can lead to more severe problems down the line.
- Antacids may have their place but like so much they are prescribed and purchased indiscriminately and overall may become more of a problem than a solution.
-

The Funding of Biased Science?

Can big money and good science really mix?
Only, perhaps in more philanthropic societies, where profit is not the motivation.

Back in the 1920s and 30s there was, it could be argued, a golden age of research work and understanding of nutrition. For example the B Vitamins were identified between 1912 and 1937, Vitamin D in 1922, Vitamin C was isolated and synthesised in 1932-34.

We Need More 'Obsessed and Possessed' Scientists!

Perhaps the 1920s and 30s, were the twilight years of uninfluenced research in universities. From then on there was more funding and subsequent control of universities by large companies and other entities. Commercial influence will have undoubtedly had an affect on the type of research, results and conclusions. Why would anyone commercially minded fund research to conclude that certain foods and not pills could provide well-being? This may be cynical, but many of the great scientific discoveries have been made by independent individuals, possessed and obsessed in finding answers to their own questions .

More Science Built on Poor Science

In order to do better, we must acknowledge that we have witnessed more science built on poor science, such as the development of statins based on the diet/heart hypothesis of Ancel Keys' work. In addition, with many scientific papers being produced there is a tendency to only read the summaries or abstracts. This leaves all the important quirks and caveats, and possible mistakes of the actual design of the experiments and their results buried deep in the heart of the science papers, leaving bad science to escape criticism and the real science ignored and misunderstood.

Today Archived Research is Available To All

However the loading of archived research that is now available to people all over the world has led to a considerable amount of reviewing of data. For example "Google Scholar" is worth exploring or being aware of and "PubMed" specializes in reviews of clinical research, with summaries and full technical reports. It comprises 24 million biomedical citations. Included is work conducted in 1890s-1940s by the scientific community when it was still relatively "pharmaceutical /food industry influence-free".

During this period, there was interest and understanding that food choices could strongly affect the gut, and physical and mental health. However, the pharmaceutical industry's rapid growth, over the 20th century resulted in a move away from this "unsophisticated" approach to health and was predominantly discarded by the established medical community. A lot of precious, fundamental science attributed to this period has been ignored in recent history.

"Pay The Farmer Now Or Pay The Doctor Later"
This is an expression that has become more prevalent in America recently – where they have allowed profit to dominate in so much of their farming, at the expense of quality and nutritional value of the food that is produced. Realising this, some Americans are warning that food choice is boiling down to "cheap food now or medical bills later".

Wild Recommendations
With everything seemingly in a state of flux, once again, I would love to see the UK's amazing health service lead the world in changing the nature of front line care. GP surgeries could be given a major role in nutritional advice and education and possibly even look at tailored supplementation for effective preventative care.

If doctors were more in tune with the deficiencies and toxicities that are at the root of most diseases, they could emphasize the possible underlying causes and steer patients toward self-help advice on *approved* website links for better nutrition.

Filling a Vacuum
The internet is full of medical and nutritional sites recommending all sorts of things. Some recommendations are wild and even dangerous, others are sensible. Whatever they are though, they are obviously symptomatic of a need for answers and more help than we are currently getting from our doctors in our quest for well-being.

The Formidable Advancement of Medicine
Many of the scientific advances that are being made are, in all aspects of medicine, simply fantastic. Doctors, specialists and surgeons have skills and techniques available to them that are formidable. I believe we can obtain similar bold achievements at a preventative and educational end of medicine. After all where does the word doctor come from – the Latin verb *docēre* meaning "to teach".

Food, Emotion, Discipline, Routine and Projects
Food is very much linked to emotion. There are those who like to reward themselves with food when they have achieved something. There are those who resort to food when things do not go well. The link between food and emotion is much tighter when one is still addicted to sugar. Break that link, first of all, and at least our hormones will not be working against us and we have a chance of moving forward and achieving more.

Misery, Freedom and Lists
Procrastination equals misery! Misery may lead to eating naughty things… Tackle the jobs we dislike first, then we are free to get on with the rest of our day or week with a lighter load on our shoulders.

Reflect on changes that could be made to improve the daily routine; incorporate them slowly. Take time to sit down with a notebook and keep a running list of the things that need to be done, but also a list of things to arrange to look forward to. Regularly take a moment to look up a few more tasty recipes to prepare.

Value Your Time
Place more value on your time and reassess how you spend your time. Have a project on the go that you look forward to returning to, and make sure you always have a reason to jump out of bed in the morning, even when you're 90.

Conviviality
Let us not forget this wonderful part of life as we sink deeper into the virtual world! In striving to make food "convenient", we may have lost sight of it's potential to bring together friends, family, communication, laughter, music and conviviality.

We should embrace the need to cook and eat wholesome, good food that we prepare with love and attention. Thought and consideration in the planning can make the preparation of a meal far easier than we might think. Gatherings can be more frequent if they are easy and if everyone prepares and brings a dish. It will produce meals with more variety.

A far cry from a pre-prepared meal on the sofa, in front of the TV ….

160

Chaos Of The Universe

I have often thought about the chaos in the Universe and how much of what happens is random. The fact that we have managed to create as much order as we have on our little planet is a marvel. What I'm trying to say is there is, as always, a balance between empowerment, belief that we can change and improve our health through nutrition and a pursuit of ultimate control that can take over your life and not necessarily lead to a happy existence.

I saw a couple on TV who had pursued a severe calorie restriction diet for years in order to achieve longevity but the pursuit of this goal had created the bleakest of lifestyles and they turned out to be the oldest looking 60 year olds I had ever seen! So we must try our best to eat well but be careful not to obsess and get bogged down with trying to find the ultimate way of eating because there is no 'one way'.

I believe that when we look at the money we have to spend we should prioritise, if we can, the best quality food we can afford for our family and ourselves. I hope it will be our united and informed purchasing power that will change things for the better and we must be prepared to spend if we are to maintain the quality of our food. If we opt for the cheap choices now we will pay with our health later.

…. And finally   Sugar destroys health
                    Chronic inflammation is our enemy and
                    Whole foods have magnificent power to rebuild health

Eat a good variety of fresh food
Don't be afraid of precious healthy fats
Keep moving
Nurture good sleeping habits
Moderation in all things
Manage stress and
Be happy and compassionate

Happier
Healthier
Achievers
Into Old Age

Further Recommended Reading

- Dr Martin Blaser, author of "Missing Microbes"
- Sarah Boseley, Guardian newspapers award winning Health Editor and author of "The Shape We're In: How Junk Food and Diets Are Shortening Our Lives"
- Dr Dale Bredesen, author of "The End of Alzheimers" published in 2017
- Dr Natasha Campbell McBride: Masters in Neurology and Nutrition and author of "Gut and Psychology Syndrome" and "Put Your Heart in Your Mouth"
- Ivor Cummins & Dr Jeffry Gerber "Eat Rich, Live Long" published 2018
- Dr Carolyn Dean – researcher and author "The Magnesium Miracle"
- Sally Fallon: President of the Weston A Price Foundation and author of "Nourishing Traditions" published 2009
- Dr Alessio Fasano, Italian medical doctor, pediatric gastroenterologist and researcher. Chair of Pediatrics at Harvard Medical School
- Dr Jason Fung, author of "The Complete Guide to Fasting" published 2016
- Ben Goldacre, author of "Bad Science" and "Bad Pharma"
- Dr Stephen Gundry, author of "The Plant Paradox" published 2017
- Dr Stephan Guyenet, obesity researcher, neurobiologist, and author. Bachelor of Science in biochemistry (University of Virginia) and a PhD in neurobiology (University of Washington). "Whole Health Source- Nutrition and Health Science" blog.
- Dr Zoe Harcombe, author of "The Diet Fix" published 2019
- Wardeh Harmon, author of "The Complete Idiot's Guide to Fermenting Foods"
- Patrick Holford, author of "The Optimum Nutrition Bible"
- Dr Richard Johnson, author of "The Fat Switch"
- Dr Malcolm Kendrick, author of "The Cholesterol Con" and "Doctoring Data: How to sort out medical advice from medical nonsense"
- Chris Kresser, Health researcher, author and blogger "chriskresser.com" has 250,000 followers
- Dr Robert Lustig, author of "Fat Chance" published 2014
- Chris Masterjohn PhD in Nutritional Sciences at City University of New York. Author of blog called "The Daily Lipid"
- Joseph Mercola, author of "Fat for Fuel" published 2018

- Linus Pauling Twice Nobel Prize Winner. Author of "Vitamin C and the Common Cold"
- Dr David Perlmutter: Board Certified Neurologist and Fellow of the American College of Nutrition. Author of New York Times No. 1 best seller "Grain Brain" and "Brain Maker"
- Weston A Price Foundation website
- Monica Reinagel, Masters in Human Nutrition, Board Certified nutrition specialist. Author of "The Inflammation Free Diet Plan"
- Jo Robinson, author of "Eating on the Wild Side: A radical new way to select and prepare foods to reclaim the nutrients and flavour we've lost"
- Gene Stone, New York Times No. 1 best seller author of "Forks Over Knives" and "The Secrets of People Who Never Get Sick"
- Gary Taubes, American author of Nobel Dreams, Bad Science: The Short Life and Weird Times of Cold Fusion, and Good Calories, Bad Calories, titled The Diet Delusion in the UK and Australia
- Nina Teicholz, author of "The Big Fat Surprise: Why Meat Butter and Cheese Belong in a Healthy Diet" published 2014.

REFERENCES

FOREWORD

1. Type 2 Diabetes Etiology and reversibility Roy Taylor, MD, FRCP Corresponding author: Roy Taylor, roy.taylor@ncl.ac.uk. Diabetes Care 2013 Apr; 36(4): 1047-1055. https://doi.org/10.2337/dc12-1805 http://care.diabetesjournals.org/content/36/4/1047.full

Hyperinsulinemia as an independent risk factor for ischemic heart disease

JP Després, B Lamarche, P Mauriège… - … England Journal of …, 1996 - Mass Medical Soc Background Prospective studies suggest that hyperinsulinemia may be an important risk factor for ischemic heart disease. However, it has not been determined whether plasma insulin levels are independently related to ischemic heart disease after adjustment for other risk factors, including plasma lipoprotein levels.

The emerging role of dietary fructose in obesity and cognitive decline

SE Lakhan, A Kirchgessner - Nutrition journal, 2013 - nutritionj.biomedcentral.com … How does Open Peer Review work? The emerging role of dietary fructose in obesity and cognitive decline … Intake of dietary fructose has also increased. In fact, high-fructose corn syrup (HFCS) accounts for as much as 40% of caloric sweeteners used in the United States …

GOLDEN NUGGETS THAT SHOULDN'T BE BURIED

1. Survival of the fattest: fat babies were the key to evolution of the large human brain. Comp Biochem Physiol A Mol Integr Physiol. 2003 Sep;136(1):17-26. Cunnane SC[1], Crawford MA.

Can a Shift in Fuel Energetics Explain the Beneficial Cardiorenal Outcomes in the EMPA-REG OUTCOME Study? A Unifying Hypothesis Sunder Mudaliar, Sindura Alloju and Robert R. Henry Diabetes Care 2016 Jun; dc160542. https://doi.org/10.2337/dc16-0542
What if It's All Been a Big Fat Lie? By Gary Taubes New York Times July 7, 2002

The big fat surprise: why butter, meat and cheese belong in a healthy diet

N Teicholz - 2014 - A New York Times bestseller Named one of The Economist's Books of the Year 2014 Named one of The Wall Street Journal's Top Ten Best Nonfiction Books of 2014 Kirkus Reviews Best Nonfiction Books of 2014 Forbes's Most Memorable Healthcare Book of 2014 …

1a. Ketones Suppress Brain Glucose Consumption Part of the Advances in Experimental Medicine and Biology book series (AEMB, volume 645) Authors: Joseph C. LaManna, Nicolas Salem, Michelle Puchowicz, Bernadette Erokwu, Smruta Koppaka, Chris Flask, Zhenghong Lee

1b. Dietdoctor.com

2. **Medium chain triglyceride diet reduces anxiety-like behaviors and enhances social competitiveness in rats** Author links open overlay panelFionaHollis[a]Ellen SiobhanMitchell[b]CarlesCanto[b]DongmeiWang[b]CarmenSandi[a] https://doi.org/10.1016/j.neuropharm.2018.06.017Get rights and content

2a. **Memory Enhancers** E Halevas, GK Katsipis, AA Pantazaki - Biotechnological Applications 2019 – Springer -

3. **Adipose tissue dysregulation and reduced insulin sensitivity in non-obese individuals with enlarged abdominal adipose cells.** Hammarstedt A[1], Graham TE, Kahn BB. Diabetol Metab Syndr. 2012 Sep 19;4(1):42. doi: 10.1186/1758-5996-4-42.

4. **Insulin-sensitive obesity.** Am J Physiol Endocrinol Metab. 2010 Sep;299(3):E506-15. doi: 10.1152/ajpendo.00586.2009. Epub 2010 Jun 22. Klöting N[1], Fasshauer M, Dietrich A, Kovacs P, Schön MR, Kern M, Stumvoll M, Blüher M.

5. **Kraft JR. Detection of diabetes mellitus *in situ* (occult diabetes). Lab Med 1975;6:10–22. 10.1093/labmed/6.2.10** Postprandial insulin assay as the earliest biomarker for diagnosing pre-diabetes, type 2 diabetes and increased cardiovascular risk James J DiNicolantonio,[1] Jaikrit Bhutani,[2] James H OKeefe,[1] and Catherine Crofts[3]

5a. **Insulin resistance and hyperinsulinemia: is hyperinsulinemia the cart or the horse?** *https://www.ncbi.nlm.nih.gov/pubmed/18227495* by MH Shanik - 2008 -

5b. **Hyperinsulinemia as an independent risk factor for ischemic heart disease** JP Després, B Lamarche, P Mauriège… - … England Journal of …, 1996 - Mass Medical Soc

6. **Reversing Type 2 Diabetes through diet Effectiveness and safety of a novel care model for the management of type 2 diabetes at 1 year: an open-label, non-randomized, controlled study** SJ Hallberg, AL McKenzie, PT Williams, NH Bhanpuri… - Diabetes Therapy, 2018 **Cardiovascular disease risk factor responses to a type 2 diabetes care model including nutritional ketosis induced by sustained carbohydrate restriction at 1year.** NH Bhanpuri, SJ Hallberg… - Cardiovascular …, 2018 - cardiab.biomedcentral.com **A novel intervention including individualized nutritional recommendations reduces hemoglobin A1c level, medication use, and weight in type 2 diabetes** AL McKenzie, SJ Hallberg, BC Creighton, BM Volk… - … Diabetes, 2017 - diabetes.jmir.org **Dr. Sarah Hallberg** is the medical director and founder of the Indiana University-Arnett Health Medical Weight Loss Program. She created the program around 2012 and since then it has helped hundreds of patients reverse and prevent type 2 diabetes through low carb and high fat nutrition. http://www.diabetes.co.uk/blog/2015/05/ignore-the-guidelines-eat-low-carb-and-high-fat-dr-sarah-hallberg-on-how-to-reverse-type-two-diabetes/

Proquest **Carbohydrates, Insulin, and Obesity.** Scherger, Joseph E.**Internal Medicine Alert; Atlanta** Vol. 40, Iss. 20, (Oct 2018). SOURCE : **Astley CM, Todd JN, Salem RM, et al. Genetic evidence that carbohydrate-stimulated insulin secretion leads to obesity.** *Clin Chem* **2018:64:192-200.**

7. **Hyperinsulinemia as an Independent Risk Factor for Ischemic Heart Disease**
Jean-Pierre Després, Ph.D., Benoît Lamarche, M.Sc., Pascale Mauriège, Ph.D., Bernard Cantin, M.D., Gilles R. Dagenais, M.D., Sital Moorjani, Ph.D., and Paul-J. Lupien, M.D.
April 11, 1996 N Engl J Med 1996; 334:952-958 DOI: 10.1056/NEJM199604113341504

8. Survival of the fattest: fat babies were the key to evolution of the large human brain. **PubMed.gov Comp Biochem Physiol A Mol Integr Physiol. 2003 Sep;136(1):17-26. Cunnane SC[1], Crawford MA.**

9. Fructose consumption as a risk factor for non-alcoholic fatty liver disease *
Xiaosen Ouyang[1, †], Pietro Cirillo[1], Yuri Sautin[1], Shannon McCall[2], James L. Bruchette[2], Anna Mae Diehl[3], Richard J. Johnson[1], Manal F. Abdelmalek[3, ·]

"The role of fructose in the pathogenesis of NAFLD and the metabolic syndrome" Jung Sub Lim, Michele Mietus-Snyder, Annie Valente, Jean-Marc Schwarz & Robert H. Lustig
http://www.nature.com/nrgastro/journal/v7/n5/full/nrgastro.2010.41.html

Dr R Lustig "Fat Chance" Published by Fourth Estate in October 2014

10. **Addiction To Fructose - The Addiction Potential of Hyperpalatable Foods**
http://www.ingentaconnect.com/content/ben/cdar/2011/00000004/00000003/art00003
Authors: N. Gearhardt, Ashley; Davis, Caroline; Kuschner, Rachel; D. Brownell, Kelly
http://www.sciencedirect.com/science/article/pii/S0149763407000589
Science Direct Elsevier Neuroscience & Biobehavioral ReviewsVolume 32, Issue 1, 2008, Pages 20–39 Authors Nicole M. Avena, Pedro Rada, Bartley G. Hoebel
Evidence for sugar addiction: Behavioral and neurochemical effects of intermittent, excessive sugar intake Avena, N.M., Rada, P., Hoebel B.G., 2007.

11. **Advanced glycation end products. Key players in skin ageing?** Paraskevi Gkogkolou and Markus Böhm· Dermatoendocrinol. 2012 Jul 1; 4(3): 259–270.
doi: 10.4161/derm.22028 PMCID: PMC3583887 PMID: 23467327

12. Hyperinsulinemia: a Cause of Obesity? - NCBI – NIH
https://www.ncbi.nlm.nih.gov/pmc/articles/PMC5487935/ by KA Erion - 2017 -
2 May 2017 - The recent emergence of the concept of selective insulin resistance, in which tissues become resistant to insulin's effect on glucose transport but remain sensitive to its lipogenic effect, has reinvigorated the hypothesis that HI may be a primary cause of weight gain that leads to obesity and type 2 diabetes

Chapter 1

1. Food as Exposure: Nutritional Epigenetics and the New Metabolism
http://www.palgrave-journals.com/biosoc/journal/v6/n2/full/biosoc20111a.html
Dr D Perlmutter – Brain Maker Published by Little, Brown and Company April 2015
2. Dr Zoe Harcombe WHO study of cholesterol and death from heart disease and all cause mortality.
3. Dr Joseph Kraft "Diabetes Epidemic and You" Published 2008

Chapter 3

1. A review of fatty acid profiles and antioxidant ... - Nutrition Journal
https://nutritionj.biomedcentral.com/articles/10.1186/1475-2891-9-10
by CA Daley - 2010 - Cited by 566 - Related articles
10 Mar 2010 - Research spanning three decades suggests that grass-based diets can significantly improve the fatty acid (FA) composition and antioxidant ...

1a. Metabolic characteristics of keto-adapted ultra-endurance runners

JS Volek, DJ Freidenreich, C Saenz, LJ Kunces… - Metabolism, 2016 - Elsevier
Background Many successful ultra-endurance athletes have switched from a high-carbohydrate to a low-carbohydrate diet, but they have not previously been studied to determine the extent of metabolic adaptations. Methods Twenty elite ultra-marathoners and …

1b. See the work of Dr Stephen Cunnane on brain glucose and ketone metabolism. PhD in Physiology from McGill University and completed post-doctoral research on nutrition and brain development. He has researched fatty acids and their effect on brain development as well as the effect of ketones and ketogenic diets on brain development. He has published over 280 peer-reviewed research papers.
Introduction: Deteriorating brain glucose metabolism precedes the clinical onset of Alzheimer's disease (AD) and appears to contribute to its etiology. Ketone ... Croteau et al. AD MCI CMR Exper Gerontol 2017 – IHMC *https://www.ihmc.us/.../uploads/.../Croteau-et-al.-AD-MCI-CMR-Exper-Gerontol-201...by E Croteau - 2017 -*
Brain fuel metabolism, ageing, and Alzheimer's disease. Stephen C. Cunnane, S. Nugent,+14 *authors Stanley I. Rapoport Published 2011 in Nutrition DOI:10.1016/j.nut.2010.07.021*
A Dual Tracer PET-MRI Protocol for the Quantitative Measure of Regional Brain Energy Substrates Uptake in the Rat J Vis Exp. 2013; (82): 50761. Published online 2013 Dec 28. doi: 10.3791/50761. PMCID: PMC4106370 PMID: 24430432 Maggie Roy, [1] Scott Nugent, [1] Sébastien Tremblay, [2] Maxime Descoteaux, [3] Jean-François Beaudoin, [2] Luc Tremblay, [2] Roger Lecomte, [2,4] and Stephen C Cunnane [1]

2. A ketogenic diet favorably affects serum biomarkers for cardiovascular disease in normal-weight men…, AL Gómez, TP Scheett, JS Volek - The Journal of …, 2002 - academic.oup.com

A review of low-carbohydrate ketogenic diets
…, J Mavropoulos, WS Yancy, JS Volek - Current atherosclerosis …, 2003 - Springer

Cardiovascular and hormonal aspects of very-low carbohydrate ketogenic diets
JS Volek, MJ Sharman - Obesity research, 2004 - Wiley Online Library

Low-carbohydrate nutrition and metabolism⁻
…, JC Mavropoulos, MC Vernon, JS Volek… - … American journal of …, 2007 - academic.oup.com

Carbohydrate restriction has a more favorable impact on the metabolic syndrome than a low fat diet
JS Volek, SD Phinney, CE Forsythe, EE Quann… - Lipids, 2009 - Springer

Carbohydrate restriction improves the features of Metabolic Syndrome. Metabolic Syndrome may be defined by the response to carbohydrate restriction JS Volek, RD Feinman - Nutrition & metabolism, 2005 - nutritionandmetabolism … Metabolic Syndrome (MetS) represents a constellation of markers that indicates a predisposition to diabetes, cardiovascular disease and other pathologic states. The definition and treatment are a matter of current debate and there is not general agreement …

3. Fat For Fuel by Dr Joseph Mercola published 2017

Chapter 4

1. Demographics, Risk Factors and Outcomes of Stroke in Young Adults Aged 18-45 Years in Comparison With Those Older Than 45 Years
N Nagaraja, S Jugl, JD Brown, AN Simpkins… - Stroke, 2019 - Am Heart Assoc

2. Eat Rich Live Long by Ivor Cummins and Dr Jeffry Gerber Published in 2018

3. You Tube Lecture – Ivor Cummins – The Pathways of Insulin Resistance: Exposure and Implications (Low Carb Down Under) 9 June 2017

Chapter 5

1. How to fix your broken metabolism by doing the exact opposite -
…https://www.dietdoctor.com/fix-broken-metabolism-exact-opposite

2. Ketogenic Medium Chain Triglycerides Increase Brain Energy Metabolism in Alzheimer's Disease. J Alzheimers Dis. 2018;64(2):551-561. doi: 10.3233/JAD-180202.
Croteau E[1], Castellano CA[1], Richard MA[2], Fortier M[1], Nugent S[3], Lepage M[2], Duchesne S[3,4], Whittingstall K[5], Turcotte ÉE[2], Bocti C[6], Fülöp T[1,6], Cunnane SC[1,6].
CONCLUSION: Ketones from MCT compensate for the brain glucose deficit in AD in direct proportion to the level of plasma ketones achieved.

3. *Inverse relationship between brain glucose and ketone metabolism in adults during short-term moderate dietary ketosis: A dual tracer quantitative positron emission tomography study…* Courchesne-Loyer et al PET KD JCBFM 2016

Chapter 6

1. Intake of saturated and trans unsaturated fatty acids and risk of all cause mortality, cardiovascular disease, and type 2 diabetes: systematic review and meta ...RJ De Souza, A Mente, A Maroleanu, AI Cozma, V Ha... - Bmj, 2015 - bmj.com Objective To systematically review associations between intake of saturated fat and trans unsaturated fat and all cause mortality, cardiovascular disease (CVD) and associated mortality, coronary heart disease (CHD) and associated mortality, ischemic stroke, and type 2 diabetes. Design Systematic review and meta-analysis. Data sources Medline, Embase,

2. **Food consumption and the actual statistics of cardiovascular diseases ...**
https://foodandnutritionresearch.net/index.php/fnr/article/view/982 by P Grasgruber - 2016 -

27 Sep 2016 - Pavel **Grasgruber** Faculty of Sports Studies Masaryk University, Brno Czech ...

consumption of animal fat and animal protein (r=0.92, **p**<0.001).

Conclusion: Our results do not support the association between CVDs and saturated fat, which is still contained in official dietary guidelines. Instead, they agree with data accumulated from recent studies that link CVD risk with the high glycaemic index/load of carbohydrate-based diets. In the absence of any scientific evidence connecting saturated fat with CVDs, these findings show that current dietary recommendations regarding CVDs should be seriously reconsidered.

3. **The association between dietary saturated fatty acids and ischemic**
https://www.ncbi.nlm.nih.gov/pubmed/26791181 by J Praagman - 2016

4. **Associations of fats and carbohydrate intake with cardiovascular disease and mortality in 18 countries from five continents (PURE): a prospective cohort study M Dehghan**, A Mente, X Zhang, S Swaminathan, W Li... - The Lancet, 2017 – Elsevier ...

5. **A review of fatty acid profiles and antioxidant content in grass-fed and grain-fed beef**
CA Daley, A Abbott, PS Doyle... - Nutrition ..., 2010 - nutritionj.biomedcentral.com Growing consumer interest in grass-**fed** beef products has raised a number of questions with regard to the perceived differences in nutritional quality between grass-**fed** and **grain-fed cattle**.

6. **"Dietary fat guidelines have no evidence base: where next for public health nutritional advice?" Dr Zoe Harcombe et al.** Published in the British Journal of Sports Medicine 2016.

7. **Other reviews of the evidence that conclude that dietary fat guidelines have no evidence base**: Skeaff & Miller 2009 / Siri-Tarino et al 2010 / Hooper et al 2011 / Chowdhury et al 2014 / Schwingshackl & Hoffman 2014 / Hooper et al 2015

8. **Dr Z Harcombe Parliamentary address** – YouTube video https://youtu.be/IQVsHtPUUQI

Chapter 7

1. Regulatory T-cell homeostasis: steady-state maintenance ... - NCBI - NIH
https://www.ncbi.nlm.nih.gov/pubmed/24712458 by KS Smigiel - 2014 -
Immunol Rev. 2014 May;259(1):40-59. doi: 10.1111/imr.12170. Regulatory T-cell homeostasis: steady-state maintenance and modulation during inflammation.

1a. **Inflammation Cause Of Many Modern Diseaseswww**.cdc.gov/pcd/issues/2012/11_0301.htm
by G Egger - 2012 - This focus on a predominant cause of infections (ie, microbial pathogens)

ultimately led to ... The discovery of a form of low-grade systemic and chronic inflammation ... for many developed countries; approximately 70% of diseases now result from ... These include not only behaviors linked to modern lifestyles facilitated by ...

Chapter 8

1. Omega 6 And Inflammation www.ncbi.nlm.nih.gov/pubmed/12442909
The importance of the ratio of omega-6/omega-3 essential fatty acids. by AP Simopoulos - 2002
The Center for Genetics, Nutrition and Health, Washington, DC 20009, USA. cgnh@bellatlantic.net
Excessive amounts of omega-6 polyunsaturated fatty acids (PUFA) and a very ... cardiovascular disease, cancer, and inflammatory and autoimmune diseases, ...
umm.edu/health/medical/altmed/supplement/omega6-fatty-acids 20 Jun 2013

1a. Changes in consumption of omega-3 and omega-6 fatty acids in the United States during the 20th century
Tanya L Blasbalg, Joseph R Hibbeln, Christopher E Ramsden, Sharon F Majchrzak, Robert R Rawlings Am J Clin Nutr. 2011 May; 93(5): 950–962. Published online 2011 Mar
2. doi: 10.3945/ajcn.110.006643 PMCID: PMC3076650

2. Dangers Of Trans Fats "Mar 8 2014 FDA filing by HARVARD SCHOOL OF PUBLIC HEALTH – on the Tentative Determination Regarding Partially Hydrogenated Oils; Request for Comments and for Scientific Data and Information"..

3. Polyunsaturated fatty acids and inflammation
PC Calder - Prostaglandins, leukotrienes and essential fatty acids, 2006 - Elsevier
… Long chain n-3 PUFAs from oily fish and fish **oils** decrease the production of **inflammatory** … and long-term supplementation with fish **oil** on the incorporation of n-3 **polyunsaturated** fatty acids … and interleukin 1β production of diets enriched in n-3 fatty acids from **vegetable oil** or fish …

3a. Dietary omega-6 fatty acid lowering increases bioavailability of omega-3 polyunsaturated fatty acids in human plasma lipid pools
Ameer Y. Taha, Yewon Cheon, Keturah F. Faurot, Beth MacIntosh, Sharon F. Majchrzak-Hong, J. Douglas Mann, Joseph R. Hibbeln, Amit Ringel, Christopher E. Ramsden
Prostaglandins Leukot Essent Fatty Acids. Author manuscript; available in PMC 2015 May 1. Published in final edited form as: Prostaglandins Leukot Essent Fatty Acids. 2014 May; 90(5): 151–157. Published online 2014 Feb 24. doi: 10.1016/j.plefa.2014.02.003 PMCID: PMC4035030

4. Demonization Of Butter
Point 1. en.wikipedia.org/wiki/Crisco
Crisco is a brand of shortening produced by The J.M. Smucker Company popular in the United States. Introduced in June 1911 by Procter & Gamble,

5. The Questionable Link Between Saturated Fat and Heart ...
www.wsj.com/.../SB10001424052702303678404579533760760481486 6 May 2014 - Our distrust of saturated fat can be traced back to the 1950s, to a man named Ancel Benjamin Keys, a scientist at the University of Minnesota.

6. "Bad Science" and "Bad Pharma" Books by Ben Goldacre

November 21st, 2009 The Guardian by Ben Goldacre in bad science, big pharma, ... known as
The Seven Countries study, where Ancel Keys disregarded all of the countries ...

7. Saturated Fat Raises Hdl J Clin Invest. 1993 Apr; 91(4): 1665–1671.doi: 10.1172/JCI116375
Dietary fat increases high density lipoprotein (HDL) levels both by increasing the transport rates and decreasing the fractional catabolic rates of HDL cholesterol ester and apolipoprotein (Apo) A-I. Presentation of a new animal model and mechanistic studies in human Apo A-I transgenic and control mice.T Hayek, Y Ito, N Azrolan, R B Verdery, K Aalto-Setälä, A Walsh, and J L Breslow

8. SATURATED FATS – ANXIETY, MOOD SWINGS AND VIOLENCE
Trans Fat Consumption and Aggression - NCBI – NIH
https://www.ncbi.nlm.nih.gov/pmc/articles/PMC3293881/ **by BA Golomb - 2012 -** Related articles 5
Mar 2012 - A prior study looked at trans and saturated fats on depression; we ..... Intensification of essential fatty acid deficiency in the rat by dietary trans fatty acids. .... Golomb BA, Stattin H, Mednick S. Low cholesterol and violent crime.
Assessing the Observed Relationship between Low Cholesterol and Violence-related Mortality Implications for Suicide Risk. Jay R. Kaplan, Stephen B. Manuck And J. John Mann Article first published online: 17 DEC 2006 DOI: 10.1111/j.1749-6632.1997.tb52355.x Issue Annals of the New York Academy of Sciences Volume 836, Neurobiology of Suicide,

9. Why We Need Saturated Fat Mary Enig – Westonaprice.org **"Benefits of Saturated Fats"**
Mary Enig attended University of Maryland, College Park (UMCP) MS and PhD in Nutritional Sciences in 1984. From 1984 through 1991, faculty research associate at UMCP with the Lipids Research Group in the Department of Chemistry and Biochemistry, participated in biochemical research on lipids. Licensed Nutritionist in Maryland from May 1988 to October 2008. Master of the American College of Nutrition. and former editor of the *Journal of the American College of Nutrition* where she published articles on food fats and oils.[Board member and the vice president and of the Weston A. Price Foundation which she co-founded with Sally Fallon in 1999 to promote nutrition and health advice based on the work of early 20th century dentist and researcher Weston A. Price.[

10. SATURATED FAT ON BRAIN FUNCTION
Dr D Perlmutter – Brain Maker Published by Little, Brown and Company April 2015. Saturated Fat and Health: Recent Advances in Research Richard D. Feinman⊠ Lipids. 2010 Oct; 45(10): 891–892. Published online 2010 Sep 9. doi: 10.1007/s11745-010-3446-8 PMCID: PMC2974200

Chapter 9

1. Which Nutritional Factors Are Good for HDL? - ResearchGate
https://www.researchgate.net/.../328605716
2 Jan 2019 - [15] and **consumption of various fatty acids** [16], on **serum. HDL-C** levels. ... The summary of **effects** of nutritional factors on **HDL-C**. and other ...
Effects of Consumption of Various Fatty Acids on Serum ... We previously studied **effects of intake of various** dietary fat on **serum HDL-C** levels to ..... Journal of Endocrinology and Metabolism is published by **Elmer Press** Inc 21 Sep 2018 - .
https://www.jofem.org/index.php/jofem/article/view/534/284284328
by H Yanai - 2018

1a.www.cholesterolcode.com Dave Feldman

1b.High cholesterol may protect against infections and atherosclerosis
U. Ravnskov *Q.IM· An International Journal of Medicine*, Volume 96, Issue 12, 1 December 2003, Pages 927–934, https://doi.org/10.1093/qjmed/hcg150

2. Three Reasons to Abandon Low-Density Lipoprotein Targets
https://www.ahajournals.org/doi/pdf/10.1161/CIRCOUTCOMES.111.964676
by RA Hayward - 2012 - Cited by 145 - Related articles
Three Reasons to Abandon Low-Density ... density lipoprotein (LDL) cholesterol levels. ATP III ... approach, a step that could launch a new era of guidelines in.

3. Newly detected abnormal glucose tolerance: an important ... - NCBI
https://www.ncbi.nlm.nih.gov/pubmed/15541834 by M Bartnik - 2004 - Cited by 413 - Related articles
Newly detected abnormal glucose tolerance: an important predictor of long-term outcome after ... Bartnik M(1), Malmberg K, Norhammar A, Tenerz A, Ohrvik J, Rydén L. ... All patients who died from cardiovascular causes had abnormal GT.

4. Relations between metabolic syndrome, oxidative stress and inflammation and cardiovascular disease P Holvoet - Verh K Acad Geneeskd Belg, 2008 - researchgate.net The metabolic syndrome is a common and complex disorder combining obesity, dyslipidemia, hypertension, and insulin resistance.(1-4) It is a primary risk factor for diabetes and cardiovascular disease (5-13). About 80% of all type 2 diabetes is associated with …

5. Relation of circulating oxidized LDL to obesity and insulin ... - NCBI - NIH
https://www.ncbi.nlm.nih.gov/pubmed/20102528 by AS Kelly - 2010
Pediatr Diabetes. 2010 Dec;11(8):552-5. doi: 10.1111/j.1399-5448.2009.00640.x .

Chapter 10

1. Increase in sugar consumption
http://wholehealthsource.blogspot.co.uk/2012/02/by-2606-us-diet-will-be-100-percent.html
Stephan Guyenet Obesity researcher, neurobiologist, and author. BS in biochemistry (University of Virginia) and a PhD in neurobiology (University of Washington).

2. Metabolic Syndrome
www.ncbi.nlm.nih.gov/pubmed/17921363
by RJ Johnson - 2007 - Cited by 491 - Related articles
Potential role of sugar (fructose) in the epidemic of hypertension, obesity and the metabolic syndrome, diabetes, kidney disease, and cardiovascular disease. ... may be a major mechanism by which fructose can cause cardiorenal disease.

3. Sugar, Fructose, Fruit – Sorting Out The Confusion
http://www.nature.com/nrgastro/journal/v7/n5/full/nrgastro.2010.41.html
"The role of fructose in the pathogenesis of NAFLD and the metabolic syndrome" Jung Sub Lim, Michele Mietus-Snyder, Annie Valente, Jean-Marc Schwarz & Robert H. Lustig

Dr R Lustig "Fat Chance" Published by Fourth Estate in October 2014
"A causal role for uric acid in fructose-induced metabolic syndrome"
Takahiko Nakagawa, Hanbo Hu, Sergey Zharikov, Katherine R. Tuttle, Robert A. Short, Olena Glushakova, Xiaosen Ouyang, Daniel I. Feig, Edward R. Block, Jaime Herrera-Acosta, Jawaharlal M. Patel, Richard J. Johnson
American Journal of Physiology - Renal Physiology Published 1 March 2006 Vol. 290 no. 3, F625-F631 DOI: 10.1152/ajprenal.00140.2005 http://ajprenal.physiology.org/content/290/3/F625.short

4. Fat Storage System Hibernating bear / Fat Storage System
http://www.ncbi.nlm.nih.gov/pmc/articles/PMC3660463/ Dr R Johnson

5. Fructose Does Not Suppress Ghrelin www.ncbi.nlm.nih.gov/pubmed/15181085
by KL Teff - 2004 - Cited by 496 - Related articles Because fructose, unlike glucose, does not stimulate insulin secretion, we ... but postprandial suppression of ghrelin was significantly less pronounced after HFr ...

6. Fructose Suppresses The I'm Full Signal Peptide Yy "Dietary Sugars and Health" Edited by Michael I Goran, Luc Tappy, Kim-Anne Le. CRC Press Taylor and Francis Group page 198

7. Fructose Suppresses Leptin www.ncbi.nlm.nih.gov/pubmed/15181085 by KL Teff - 2004 - Dietary fructose reduces circulating insulin and leptin, attenuates postprandial suppression of ghrelin, and increases triglycerides in women. Teff KL(1), Elliott SS ...

ADDITIONAL REFERENCES FOR SUGAR AND DISEASE
UCSF Mini Medical School for the Public UCTV **Childhood Obesity: Adrift in the "Limbic Triangle"** Michelle L. Mietus-Snyder and Robert H. Lustig *Annual Review of Medicine* 59:147-162 (February 2008)
Childhood Obesity: Behavioral Aberration or Biochemical Drive? Reinterpreting the First Law of Thermodynamics Robert H. Lustig*Nature Clinical Practice Endocrinology & Metabolism* 2(8):447-458 (2006)
Adolescent Overweight and Future Adult Coronary Heart Disease
Kirsten Bibbins-Domingo, Pamela Coxson, Mark T. Pletcher, James Lightwood and Lee Goldman *New England Journal of Medicine*, 357(23):2371-2379 (Dec. 6, 2007)
Overweight Adolescents Projected to Have More Heart Disease in Young Adulthood
UCSF News Release, Dec. 5, 2007
Prevalence of Overweight and Obesity in the United States, 1999-2004
Cynthia L. Ogden, Margaret D. Carroll, Lester R. Curtin, Margaret A. McDowell, Carolyn J. Tabak and Katherine M. Flegal *JAMA*, 295(13):1549-1555 (April 5, 2006)

8. Fructose On The Liver Journal of Hepatology Volume 48, Issue 6, June 2008, Pages 993-999
Ref: Effects of sucrose, glucose and fructose on peripheral and central appetite signals. Dept of Experimental Medical Science, Lund University, Lund Sweden 2007 A Lindqvist et al

9. Fructose and Vitamin D. Ref: Dietary fructose inhibits intestinal calcium absorption and induces vitamin D insufficiency in CKD. Journal of the American Society of Nephrology 21 (2), 261-271, 2010.

10. **Why Sweeteners Are Not A Good Idea** http://blogs.scientificamerican.com/mind-guest-blog/tricking-taste-buds-but-not-the-brain-artificial-sweeteners-change-braine28099s-pleasure-response-to-sweet/ Tricking Taste Buds but Not the Brain: Artificial Sweeteners Change Brain's Pleasure Response to Sweet

11. **It's Not The Fat – It's The Sugar** 2010 American Society for Nutrition Meta-analysis of prospective cohort studies evaluating the association of saturated fat with cardiovascular disease[1,2,3,4,5] Patty W Siri-Tarino, Qi Sun, Frank B Hu, and Ronald M Krauss Author Affiliations From the Children's Hospital Oakland Research Institute Oakland CA (PWS TRMK)the Departments of Nutrition (QSFBH)Epidemiology (FBH) Harvard School of Public Health Boston MA.

Chapter 12

1. **Deodorization** - AOCS lipidlibrary.aocs.org/OilsFats/content.cfm?ItemNumber=40326 27 Jan 2014

Chapter 13   IGNORING THE MICROBIOME

1. **"Missing Microbes" Author: Dr Martin Blaser**

2. http://www.actionbioscience.org/genomics/the_human_microbiome.html
Dr D Perlmutter – **Brain Maker** Published by Little, Brown and Company April 2015
The Economist magazine of August 18, 2012 **The human microbiome Me, myself, us**
http://www.sciencedirect.com/science/article/pii/S0165247804000379
Commensal bacteria (normal microflora), mucosal immunity and chronic inflammatory and autoimmune diseases
http://genome.cshlp.org/content/19/12/2317 The NIH Human Microbiome Project

3. **Gut/Brain Axis**
"**Gut and Psychology Syndrome**" Author: Dr Natasha Campbell McBride MD MMedSci (neurology), MMedSci (nutrition).
Li, W.; Dowd, S. E.; Scurlock, B.; Acosta-Martinez, V.; Lyte, M. (2009).
"**Memory and learning behavior in mice is temporally associated with diet-induced alterations in gut bacteria**". *Physiology & Behavior* 96 (4–5): 557–567. doi:10.1016/j.physbeh.2008.12.004. PMID 19135464.
"**Gastrointestinal Microflora Studies in Late-Onset Autism**". *Clinical Infectious Diseases* 35 (Suppl 1): S6–S16. doi:10.1086/341914. PMID 12173102. Finegold, S. M.; Molitoris, D.; Song, Y.; Liu, C.; Vaisanen, M. L.; Bolte, E.; McTeague, M.; Sandler, R.; Wexler, H.; Marlowe, E. M.; Collins, M. D.; Lawson, P. A.; Summanen, P.; Baysallar, M.; Tomzynski, T. J.; Read, E.; Johnson, E.; Rolfe, R.; Nasir, P.; Shah, H.; Haake, D. A.; Manning, P.; Kaul, A. (2002).
"**Reduced anxiety-like behavior and central neurochemical change in germ-free mice**". *Neurogastroenterology & Motility* 23 (3): 255–264, e119. doi:10.1111/j.1365-2982.2010.01620.x. PMID 21054680. Neufeld, K. M.; Kang, N.; Bienenstock, J.; Foster, J. A. (2011).

4. **Prescriptions For Asthma** asthma research council http://www.asthma.org.uk/history

5. **Caesarian Sections** "Missing Microbes" Author: Dr Martin Blaser Chapter 9 "Mother and Child"

6. The Most Significant Contribution To Gut Health Is Believed To Be Fibre From Whole Plant Foods And Polyphenols http://pubs.acs.org/doi/abs/10.1021/jf2053959 Up-regulating the Human Intestinal Microbiome Using Whole Plant Foods, Polyphenols, and/or Fiber http://www.phenol-explorer.eu http://www.ncbi.nlm.nih.gov/pubmed/24452238

Am J Clin Nutr. 2014 Mar;99(3):479-89. doi: 10.3945/ajcn.113.074237. Epub 2014 Jan 22. Flavonoid-rich fruit and vegetables improve microvascular reactivity and inflammatory status in men at risk of cardiovascular disease--FLAVURS: a randomized controlled trial. Macready AL1, George TW, Chong MF, Alimbetov DS, Jin Y, Vidal A, Spencer JP, Kennedy OB, Tuohy KM, Minihane AM, Gordon MH, Lovegrove JA; FLAVURS Study Group.

7. C Difficile And Fecal Transplants "Missing Microbes" Author: Dr Martin Blaser

8. Firmicutes And Bacteriodetes http://www.pnas.org/content/107/33/14691.long

Impact of diet in shaping gut microbiota revealed by a comparative study in children from Europe and rural Africa

9. Altering Your Ratio

http://www.researchgate.net/profile/George_Fahey/publication/269876705_Fiber_supplementation_influences_phylogenetic_structure_and_functional_capacity_of_the_human_intestinal_microbiome_follow-up_of_a_randomized_controlled_trial/links/54aab4410cf25c4c472f484a.pdf

10. The Microbiome And Our Genes 23,000 genes – 3million genes The Economist magazine of August 18, 2012 The human microbiome http://www.ncbi.nlm.nih.gov/pmc/articles/PMC3764083/ The Environment Within: Exploring the Role of the Gut Microbiome in Health and Disease Environ Health Perspect. 2013 Sep; 121(9): A276–A281.

11. Caution And Balance And A New Type Of Medicine Chapter 9 – A Forgotten World from "Missing Microbes – How Killing Bacteria Creates Modern Plagues" by Martin Blaser. Published by One World

12. War Probiotics And Their Fermented Food Products Are Beneficial For Health.

Https://Www.Ncbi.Nlm.Nih.Gov/Pubmed/16696665 By S Parvez - 2006

Parvez S(1), Malik KA, Ah Kang S, Kim HY. Author Information: (1)Helix Pharms Co. Ltd, Kyung-Hee University, And Department Of Biological Sciences Of Oriental Medicine, Graduate School Of Interdepartmental Studies, Institute Of Oriental Medicines, Kyung-Hee University, Dongdaemoon-Gu, Seoul, Korea. Probiotics Are ..

Chapter 14 SPOTLIGHT ON PHYTONUTRIENTS

1. Spotlight On Polyphenol Phytonutrients And The Benefits Of Plant Foods

2004 American Society for Clinical Nutrition Polyphenols: food sources and bioavailability Claudine Manach, Augustin Scalbert, Christine Morand, Christian Rémésy, and Liliana Jiménez

2. Top Tip To Make You Tip Top http://www.ncbi.nlm.nih.gov/pubmed/11087546

J Agric Food Chem. 2000 Nov;48(11):5731-5. Differential inhibition of human platelet aggregation by selected Allium thiosulfinates. Briggs WH1, Xiao H, Parkin KL, Shen C, Goldman IL.

3. Herbs And Spices Whfoods - Carlsen MH, Halvorsen BL, Holte K et al. The total antioxidant content of more than 3100 foods, beverages, spices, herbs and supplements used worldwide.

Nutrition Journal 2010, 9:3 (22 January 2010). 2010
4. Juicing Or Blending
Mol Nutr Food Res. 2010 Nov;54(11):1646-58. doi: 10.1002/mnfr.200900580. Nonextractable polyphenols, usually ignored, are the major part of dietary polyphenols: a study on the Spanish diet. Arranz S1, Silván JM, Saura-Calixto F. PMID: 20540148 [PubMed - indexed for MEDLINE] http://nutritionfacts.org/video/juicing-removes-more-than-just-fiber/
Polyphenols as dietary fiber associated compounds. Comparative study on in vivo and in vitro properties Laura Bravo, Rocio Abia, Fulgencio Saura-Calixto *J. Agric. Food Chem.*, 1994, *42* (7), pp 1481–1487 DOI: 10.1021 /jf00043a017 Publication Date: July 1994

.

Chapter 18 ALL DISEASE IS CAUSED BY DEFICIENCY OR TOXICITY
1. The Magnesium – Calcium Relationship Is Important
http://www.nutritionalmagnesium.org/calcium-magnesium-balance/
2. "The Healing Factor" Vitamin C
IRWIN STONE (1907–1984) was an American biochemist, chemical engineer, and author of
3. VITAMIN D http://onlinelibrary.wiley.com/doi/10.1111/php.12382/full
Vitamin D and Skin Cancer - Burns - 2014 - Photochemistry and Photobiology - Wiley Online Library
4. Dietary Intake of Menaquinone Is Associated with a Reduced Risk of Coronary Heart Disease: The Rotterdam Study Johanna M. Geleijnse[*,†],Cees Vermeer[**],Diederick E. Grobbee[‡],Leon J. Schurgers[**],Marjo H. J. Knapen[**],Irene M. van der Meer[*], Albert Hofman[*], and Jacqueline C. M. Witteman[*,2] VITAMIN K2 http://jn.nutrition.org/content/134/11/3100.long
Dr. Kate Rhéaume-Bleue author of "The Calcium Paradox"

Chapter 15
1. Potential Synergies of β-Hydroxybutyrate and Butyrate on the Modulation of Metabolism, Inflammation, Cognition, and General Health.
https://www.hindawi.com/journals/jnme/2018/7195760/ by F Cavaleri - 2018 - 28 Feb 2018 -

Chapter 16
1. Do dietary lectins cause disease? - NCBI – NIH
https://www.ncbi.nlm.nih.gov/pmc/articles/PMC1115436/ by DLJ Freed - 1999
The mucus stripping effect of lectins[16] also offers an explanation for the anecdotal finding of many allergists that a "stone age diet," which eliminates most starchy foods and therefore most lectins, protects against common upper respiratory viral infections: without lectins in the throat the nasopharyngeal mucus ...
2. Leaky gut and autoimmune diseases.
Fasano A[1]. Clin Rev Allergy Immunol. 2012 Feb;42(1):71-8. doi: 10.1007/s12016-011-8291-x.

Chapter 18

1. Dr Carolyn Dean Researcher on Magnesium for 25 years and author of "The Magnesium Miracle" Revised in 2017

Chapter 19 STRESS, BABOONS AND THE BRITISH CIVIL SERVICE

1. Stress, Portrait of a Killer - Full Documentary (2008) – YouTube
https://www.youtube.com/watch?v=eYG0ZuTv5rs
The Stress and Health Study – Whitehall II Sir Michael Marmot Professor of Epidemiology and Public Health https://www.ucl.ac.uk/whitehallII University College London –

Chapter 21

1. The Weston Price Foundation Book "Nourishing Traditions" Sally Falon
Chris Masterjohn The Daily Lipid Podcasts PHD in Nutritional Sciences
1a. Diet mimicking fasting promotes regeneration and reduces ...
https://www.ncbi.nlm.nih.gov/pmc/articles/PMC4899145/ by IY Choi - 2016 - 26 May 2016 - Multiple sclerosis (MS) is an autoimmune disorder characterized by T ... Guevara- Aguirre et al., 2011; Lee et al., 2010; Longo and Mattson, 2014).
2. The modified Palaeolithic (Wahls Elimination) and low saturated fat (Swank) diets on perceived fatigue in persons with relapsing remitting multiple sclerosis …
T Wahls, MO Scott, Z Alshare, L Rubenstein… - …, 2018 - trialsjournal.biomedcentral.com
3. Low Protein Intake is Associated with a Major Reduction in IGF-1
...*https://www.ncbi.nlm.nih.gov/pmc/articles/PMC3988204/* by ME Levine - 2014 -
4. Fasano A. Leaky gut and autoimmune diseases. *Clin Rev Allergy Immunol.* 2012;42(1):71-78. doi:10.1007/s12016-011-8291-x.

Chapter 22

1. Proton-pump inhibitor therapy induces acid-related symptoms in healthy volunteers after withdrawal of therapy. Gastroenterology. 2009 Jul;137(1):80-7, 87.e1. doi: 10.1053/j.gastro.2009.03.058. Epub 2009 Apr 10. Reimer C[1], Søndergaard B, Hilsted L, Bytzer P. BACKGROUND: Rebound acid hypersecretion (RAHS) has been demonstrated after 8 weeks of treatment with a proton-pump inhibitor (PPI). If RAHS induces acid-related symptoms, this might lead to PPI dependency and thus have important implications.
2. Plasma glucose, insulin and lipid responses to high-carbohydrate low-fat diets in normal humans. Coulston AM, Liu GC, Reaven GM. Metabolism. 1983 Jan;32(1):52-6.